"Integral polarity practice is a practice rooted in c
ishing and leadership. When it comes to leaders   ___ as
love, empathy, and compassion in relation to trust,   ___vual agency, community,
and purpose establishes a compelling framework for understanding, caring for, and
motivating those we are privileged enough to lead and serve. I strongly recommend
integral polarity practice as a valuable method for bridging the gap between the inner
work essential for all leaders and the principles that pave the way for peak performance and thriving organizations."

KATY GRANVILLE-CHAPMAN DPHIL

*Co-chair the Oxford/Harvard Leadership for Flourishing Community of Practice af-
filiated with Harvard University's Human Flourishing Program at Harvard's Institute for Quantitative Social Science. Research fellow at the Oxford Character Project
and co-founder of Global Social Leaders*

"Human flourishing is defined as whole-human well-being, integrating the physical, mental, social, and moral dimensions of the human being (VanderWeele 2017).
The full expression of these dimensions includes embracing primary polar dynamics,
which can be integrated in one's awareness through stages of human development.
Giving voice to and experiencing the perspectives which arise through these polarities
and finding the stillpoint through which they can be transcended and more virtuously
expressed in support of flourishing is the very practical work of the Integral Polarity
Practice (IPP), developed by our colleague John Kesler. I have taken the IPP training
and find it helpful to understand, firsthand, how these polarities reside within me and
can be more deeply grounded in stillness, resulting in more flourishing perspectives
and engagement in the world. This acknowledging and integrating more flourishing
expression of primary polarities is a critical skillset for the multitudes taking up the
whole-human well-being of themselves and of their whole ecosystem of stakeholders,
what we call Leadership for Flourishing."

JAMES RITCHIE-DUNHAM PHD

*Clinical Associate Professor of Strategy in the Rosenthal Department of Manage-
ment at the University of Texas at Austin McCombs School of Business, lead co-editor
of Leadership for Flourishing (Oxford University Press, forthcoming), research affil-
iate of the Harvard Human Flourishing Program, department associate in the Harvard T.H. Chan School of Public Health's Social and Behavioral Sciences Department
and the Center for Work, Health, and Well-being, and president of the Institute for
Strategic Clarity.*

INTEGRAL POLARITY PRACTICE

In Service of Leadership for Flourishing

John T. Kesler

For permission requests, contact the publisher at
john@theippinstitute.com

Paperback: 979-8-9905397-0-9
Ebook: 979-8-9905397-1-6

Library of Congress Number: 2024908798

IPPI Publishing
1720 Millbrook Road
Salt Lake City, Utah 84106

theippinstitute.com

Acknowledgements

This book benefits deeply from the work of researchers, scholars, and practitioners in the Oxford/Harvard Interest Group on Leadership for Flourishing that is dedicated to reimagining leadership as empowering ecosystem wide flourishing, of which I am a member, and which is a part of the Flourishing Network at the Human Flourishing Program at Harvard University. I express particular thanks to those members of the Interest Group who reviewed the manuscript and provided endorsements and valuable feedback: Matthew T. Lee, Director of the Flourishing Network and professor at Baylor University, James Ritchie-Dunham with appointments at Harvard University and the University of Texas at Austin and president of the Institute for Strategic Clarity, and Katy Granville-Chapman, Oxford University scholar-leader and co-chair of the Interest Group.

Introduction

Over the last two decades I have developed and shared a spiritual, life, and group practice that explores timeless polarities aligned with primary qualities of our humanity and stages of human development.[1] This practice is called integral polarity practice ("IPP") and supports interrelated individual, collective, and ecosystemic flourishing. IPP is designed to complement any spiritual or belief orientation.[2] It involves practices that help us to become more centered and integrated, and over time to grow and develop so that we might live more ecosystemically flourishing lives. It can also be applied to support the work that we do to create a more flourishing world. Such internal practices and work in the world are deeply interrelated and mutually informing.

Whatever our particular philosophical orientation and organizational framework, IPP is designed to provide people and organizations with practices which support universal processes of development, flourishing, and transformation. This is particularly important in helping to guide us through the polarization and conflict that are so pervasive leading to more creative, loving, and life affirming approaches to the challenges before us.

Because we assume that the wholeness of flourishing includes the unique vision of each person to flourish and contribute in the world, and every culture and belief system to paint their own unique pictures of flourishing, the term itself is not precisely defined in IPP. However, IPP reflects some general framing assumptions about flourishing that will become evident through descriptions of the nature of IPP as a practice in this book. Here are seven of those framing assumptions:

1. Flourishing contemplates learning to become centered in stillness and spiritual depth, together with exhibiting qualities of virtuous character that arise out of that stillness and depth.
2. Flourishing includes honoring and cultivating the sacred nature of every dimension of the human being and honoring the sacred nature of all life.
3. Flourishing contemplates an endless process of connecting with and growing into the fullness of our sacred nature, which we can access within.
4. Flourishing has to do with the integration and total wellbeing of the individual, including but not limited to physical, emotional, mental, and spiritual wellbeing.
5. Love is the essence of flourishing.[3]
6. Love as the primary quality of flourishing is in intimate relationship with two other transcendent qualities of flourishing: Light and Life. Light, Love, and Life are all perhaps simply different frequencies of the same Spirit. An even deeper context for flourishing grounded in Love is appreciating the Ground or Divine Source out of which Light, Love, and Life arise and their integrated expression through a Passionate Embrace of all manifestation.
7. Flourishing of the individual is deeply interconnected with the flourishing of the collectives and ecosystems of which each of us is a part, and hence working toward full ecosystemic flourishing for all is vital.

Part 1 is a brief introduction to IPP as a practice in service of flourishing generally, which lays the groundwork for addressing the primary topic of this book in Part 2. In Part 2, I introduce how IPP can support and enhance capacities and qualities of leadership, which generate and empower more flourishing individuals and collectives of all sorts, from families to organizations, communities and global action networks, all in an ecosystemic context.

PART I

Introduction to IPP in Service of Flourishing

IPP can help you experience the pervasive presence of Love in your relationships with the Transcendent[4] (God, Divine, Spirit, Source, Ultimate, Absolute, Higher Self, Deep Stillness—however you define it[5]), with yourself, others, and our life world as the essence of flourishing. (Love in this context is a transcendent quality that draws us toward unlimited and unqualified Loving Kindness, Empathy, and Compassion.) As will be described, IPP can also help you address how to optimize flourishing through Love in the context of several interrelated, research-based principles and patterns of flourishing.

In addition, IPP can help you work with the additional aspects of flourishing and how they all interrelate and support one another including these outcomes:

- Be centered in Awakened Stillness;
- Develop loving and virtuous character;
- Be well integrated and flourishing in all dimensions of yourself;[6]
- Discover that all aspects of yourself are Sacred and honor that realization;
- Experience a transcendent aesthetic dimension to life that we call living and loving in Sacred Beauty;
- Experience ongoing personal growth, maturation, and Transformation; and
- Engage in Inspired and Creative expressions of Light, Love, and Life, through the expression of your own unique gifts.

At its core, IPP provides a framework for working with the endless polarities that we encounter in our experience. Whether we are talking about expansion and contraction, agency and communion, or countless other polarities, we define polarities as two qualities that appear to be opposites, but are complementary, and ultimately are even necessary for one another. For instance, a polar dynamic underlying our "intent" consists of moving towards something ("desire") versus moving away from something ("aversion"). Together they comprise the Intent Polarity (desire/aversion), which I explore below.

The words we use for poles of a polarity are less important than the qualities of consciousness, energy, and function that they engender. So, we use words that we have learned through facilitating IPP over the years that elicit the experience of the intended qualities most success-fully for most people, but the words do not matter as much as what we experience. Hence, the language used in the IPP polarity charts and IPP teaching and facilitation continues to evolve. As we work and train with polarities, IPP is both meditative and action-oriented in numer-ous ways, as will be explained.

Based on many years of research and facilitation, we have landed on twenty-one "Primary Polarities" selected for IPP practice that reflect primary polar dynamics central to our healthy functioning and flour-ishing through the full developmental spectrum of our humanity.[7]Nine of the Primary Polarities are functioning within us when we are born, and are designated as "Primal Polarities." Schedule 1 at the end of the book is a summary chart of the Primal Polarities. The other twelve of the Primary Polarities are designated as polarities of the "Human World," which we awaken to one by one as we grow in stages through the entire spectrum of human development. Schedule 2 is a summary chart of the Human World Polarities.

An introduction to practicing with every Primary Polarity

In IPP practice we learn how to embrace and integrate both poles of a polarity and the fields of consciousness, energy, and function that they manifest. In this process we come to realize that every aspect of our-selves is there for a good reason and is connected to a transcendent Wisdom, if we will open ourselves to it.

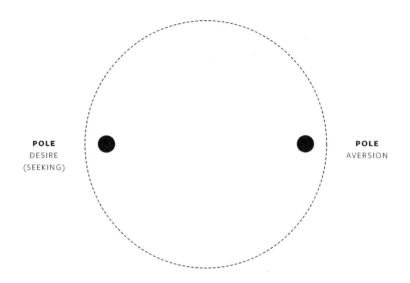

Let us look at a graphic example of an IPP polarity—the polarity of desire and aversion, which we call the Intent Polarity.

Every Primary Polarity has a Transcendent "Still Point" quality, where the polar dynamic is brought to stillness. This is accomplished by being facilitated into that stillness which will be described, and which eventually one can learn to experience on one's own. The Still Point

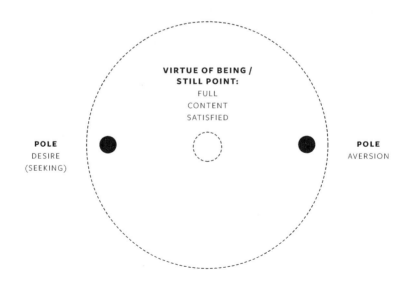

can be summarized as the Still Transcendent Essence of the bandwidth of consciousness, energy, and function represented by that polarity.[8] We call the Still Point a "Virtue of Being" because it is an experience of a still transcendent quality of "beingness." Even as the name of a given Still Point is customized to specifically bring a particular polar dynamic into Stillness, many of the experiential qualities of the Still Points of all the Primary Polarities are identical for most people, such as an experience of profound Peacefulness outside of space and time and an openness to a deeper Source of transcendent Inspiration and Love.

The Virtue of Being of each Primary Polarity naturally gives rise to a particular non-egoic, transcendent quality of attitude, called a "Virtue of Becoming" related to that polarity. In this case a deep quality of transcendent Gratitude arises out of Abundance.

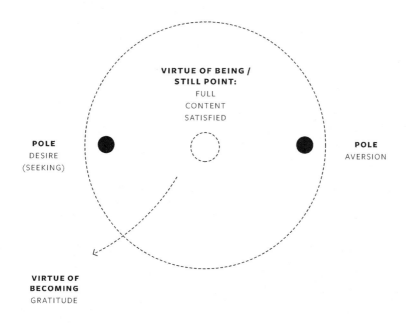

POLE
DESIRE
(SEEKING)

VIRTUE OF BEING /
STILL POINT:
FULL
CONTENT
SATISFIED

POLE
AVERSION

VIRTUE OF
BECOMING
GRATITUDE

They are called Virtues of Becoming because we are always in the process of growing into and fully integrating such transcendent qualities, even as IPP provides an immediate experience of them in their Fullness.

Each Still Point also naturally gives rise to the experience of a quality of non-egoic transcendent Engagement or "Virtue of Doing." Even though most people through IPP facilitation can access a Virtue of Doing quality within themselves, as with Virtues of Becoming, fully integrating and implementing a Virtue of Doing in our lives is likely to involve a lifetime of practice. In this case transcendent Abundance and Gratitude yield Transcendent Generosity. Transcendent Generosity is not particularly a generosity of things but rather an endless generosity of spirit.

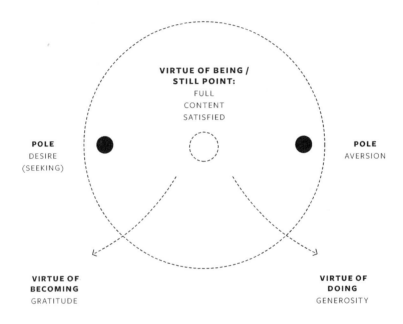

We refer to the Virtues of Becoming and Doing collectively as "Character Virtues." By practicing the Character Virtues related to a polarity, we are better able to access and deepen in the related Still Point Virtue of Being, and by learning to stabilize in the Virtue of Being, the related Character Virtues are enhanced. In short, they are all mutually informing and supportive of one another.

To flourish in the context of any particular polar dimensions of ourselves, first we have full conscious access to that aspect; second, we integrate the function of that polarity and keep it functioning and flowing freely; and third, we have stabilized in accessing and manifesting to a significant extent the Virtues of Being, Becoming, and Doing with regard to that polarity. All these steps are interrelated aspects of the flourishing of each IPP polarity, which is its own ecosystem, and which in turn contributes to our personal ecosystemic flourishing.

Note the full polarity chart on the following page for the Intent Polarity (desire/aversion). Let us explore the Intent Polarity as an example of how we frame and work with every Primary Polarity.

The Intent Polarity is the top polarity of the Primal Polarities. It transcends and yet is supported by all of them, and in that way presupposes and includes all of them. We are each born with the Intent Polarity operating within ourselves in a basic and primal way, such as having the desire to eat when hungry and to avoid pain (aversion). Even so, as we grow and develop, we ideally bring our highest awareness and capacities to make their dynamics more transparent to us. We then inform and transform these dimensions within ourselves even as these transformed dynamics in turn remain powerfully foundational to the flourishing of each of us throughout our lives. So, regarding the Intent Polarity, these qualities of desire and aversion are deeply embedded in how we address values and ideas—even our highest spiritual aspirations—as well as our most primal motivations. IPP supports us in staying consciously connected to the full spectrum of ourselves, including for example Intent Polarity dynamics, and helps bring Inspired Stewardship into what can otherwise be subconscious darkness, dysfunction, even pathology.

If we access poles of a polarity in an immature way, they function as warring opposites. In the case of the Intent Polarity there would be continual conflict between desire and aversion in many aspects of your life. The next stage of maturity is to emphasize one pole and then the other. At a further stage of maturity, both poles are present in our awareness, and they swing back and forth in an alternating cyclical way from subservience, to dominance, to subservience, etc. as each polar quality

Intention

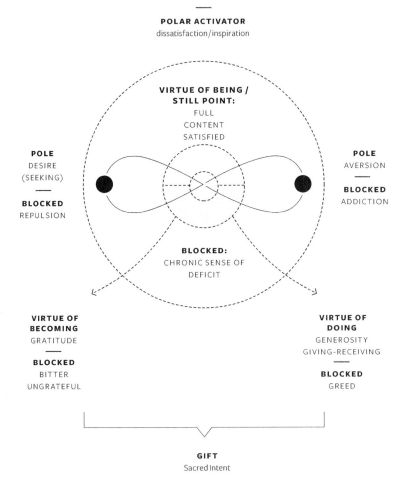

POLAR ACTIVATOR
dissatisfaction/inspiration

**VIRTUE OF BEING /
STILL POINT:**
FULL
CONTENT
SATISFIED

POLE
DESIRE
(SEEKING)

BLOCKED
REPULSION

POLE
AVERSION

BLOCKED
ADDICTION

BLOCKED:
CHRONIC SENSE OF
DEFICIT

**VIRTUE OF
BECOMING**
GRATITUDE

BLOCKED
BITTER
UNGRATEFUL

**VIRTUE OF
DOING**
GENEROSITY
GIVING-RECEIVING

BLOCKED
GREED

GIFT
Sacred Intent

needs to be balanced or emphasized in the moment.[9] The next stage of maturity is that the poles dance intimately with one another and begin to interpenetrate. This is the trajectory of maturity, with every polarity leading ultimately beyond interpenetration and finally into a Unity. Achieving this Unity results in the "polar field" being centered in a profound inner Stillness, which is that polarity's "Still Point" or "Virtue of Being."

Even if our maturity in the arena of a particular polarity has not led to a natural interpenetration and Union of the poles, most people can be facilitated into the experience of a Still Point and learn to access this experience on their own. This amounts to a "state" experience of that Unity rather than a "stage" experience, where our natural everyday experience of the polarity has matured to the point that is grounded in a stabilized deep inner Stillness. With a Primal Polarity such as desire/aversion, most of us experience a unity of intent if not a deep Stillness most of the time regarding everyday applications of intent. For example, should I pick up that pen or comb my hair in this moment? Beyond that Unity, however, IPP helps us appreciate that accessing Stillness is the key for bringing flourishing into that dimension of ourselves. For most of us, such Stillness is not a natural experience regarding applications of the polarity; we require training to attain Stillness in a profound and stabilized way.

When we experience the Still Point of the Intent Polarity, there is no deficit, nothing to desire or seek, and nothing to get away from. In IPP practice we consciously experience this Stillness in our physical dimension as Satisfaction, in our emotional and mental bandwidth as Contentment, and in the dimension of open awareness or spiritual dimension as a quality of Fullness. We sometimes summarize these qualities of this Still Point as Abundance, which also yields a profound sense of Possibility in every moment. Since most people naturally come from a place of feeling a permanent quality of deficit, being centered in this deep quality of Beingness—of Abundance—is truly transformative.

There is a paradox here because there is always a scarcity of things, or experiences that we want that we do not have, and other things that we want to get away from that burden us. For example, many of us are not as financially secure as we would like to be for ourselves and our families. However, we can learn to have a deep sense of Spiritual Abundance (Virtue of Being) in this and every moment. Initially the experience of the Still Point of a polarity is a meditative place that we access when not in the active flow of the related polar dynamics. However, the Still Point and the active quality of the polarity form their own polar relationship, which moves in the same inevitable trajectory of maturity, from a deep experience or preference for only one pole, to either/or movement, to holding both well, to interpenetration and finally a Unity. That is, regarding the dimension of intent in our lives we learn to live a flourishing life with virtuous, healthy, and well-integrated functioning of these desire/aversion polar dynamics, centered in the Stillness of these beautiful and profound interrelated qualities of Beingness: Satisfaction, Contentment, Fullness, Abundance, and Possibility.

As previously noted, the Virtue of Being of Abundance naturally generates a transcendent attitude or quality of character—a Virtue of Becoming—of Gratitude. Stabilizing in the quality of Gratitude enables us to be Grateful for every moment no matter the circumstances. In order to accomplish this, it is important to have as an aspect of our character a "Gratitude practice" to fully access, stabilize, and embed this Virtue. Even then it is a lifelong practice for most of us to fully grow into the maturity of character that fully manifests this and the rest of the IPP transcendent Virtues of Becoming.

Experiencing Abundance and Gratitude in this way naturally generates the Virtue of Doing of transcendent Generosity. This is a Generosity of Spirit, not of things. Generosity of things is limited; Generosity of Spirit is not. Just as with the Virtues of Being and Becoming, it is important to have a Generosity practice that draws on an unlimited Source through the Still Point, which can transform your life and the life of others. An example would be engaging in a Generous act of Loving Kindness beyond your normal circle of care. Through this practice, that circle of care continues to expand over time, which is an explicit indicator of deepening moral maturity.

In every Primary Polarity there is a polar dynamic that flows out of the Virtue of Doing, a pair of transcendent Polar Virtues. These Polar Virtues often seem paradoxical to the thinking mind. They nevertheless represent a deeper transcendent Logic of polar embrace. In the case of the Intent Polarity, as you will see on the chart, emerging out of Generosity is the Polar Virtue of Give/Receive. When you Give in a deep and profound way, you also Receive in a deep and profound way, and vice versa. There is, for instance, an extraordinary realization in community service work where those who are receiving support are virtually always sharing their gifts just as deeply with those who have perceived themselves to be the givers. A shared appreciation of this mutuality of Generosity generates a deep mutual Gratitude for each other in a Spirit of Abundance and Possibility.

Yet even if we have stabilized in the transcendent virtues of Abundance, Gratitude, and Generosity, there will still be challenges that will arise in this bandwidth of our consciousness, energy, and function. IPP helps us to be better prepared to deal with them. For instance, we all experience addictive tendencies related to some aspects of desire, and it is an important IPP practice to settle into Abundance and work explicitly with the polar qualities of desire/aversion that are out of balance with regard to any particular issue, such as regularly overeating, or having a consuming desire for a particular stimulant. Through IPP practice we can become aware in the moment of how desire and aversion are interacting in this context and feel the empowering influence of the inner qualities of Satisfaction, Contentment, Fullness (collectively Abundance). If we are adequately grounded in working with these polar dynamics, and coming from a place of Abundance supplemented by practicing Gratitude and Generosity, over time we can usually appropriately temper an appetite that has been out of control. Even if we need counseling or professional support to help us move beyond, for instance, an addiction or a pathological aversion to food resulting in anorexia, an IPP practice provides significant inner resources to support self-healing in this process. Many therapists trained in IPP are productively integrating IPP in their therapy for such purposes.

A remarkable realization that you find in IPP practice is that by practicing and acting through transcendent virtues such as Abundance, Gratitude, and Generosity, we discover that such transcendent qualities are already within us if we will but "wake up" to them. They seem to be ontological qualities of the Divine that are there, ready to be awakened. Rather than trying to become what we are not, we are participating in a practice that supports our growing into the Fullness of the Sacred Beings who we already are.

Also paradoxically, the Still Point of every polarity is so Full that it is Empty. That is, it is a portal to our deepest Source of Inspiration. It does not seem to matter whether you believe in a Source or the Divine or God. Each of us can experience a transcendent Influence flowing through us if we will but allow it to. This "Still Point Portal" in every IPP polarity is an opening to the Inspired and Creative non-egoic Wisdom or "Light," Unqualified and Unlimited Love, and a sense of vibrational Life-affirming qualities related in this instance to our intent.

Facilitation of Polarities

Facilitating IPP polarities is a primary modality of IPP practice. This facilitation often involves the use by the facilitator of "voice dialogue," a Jungian therapeutic technique. Through voice dialogue the facilitator speaks as and through each of the aspects of the polarities and their virtues. This is a technique that enables us to deeply experience polarities and virtues in a way that for most people is not otherwise accessible as quickly and fully.[10]

At a high level, the facilitation of a polarity through voice dialogue often looks like this:

1. A particular polarity (e.g., desire and aversion) is chosen.

2. The facilitator asks to speak to just one pole. For instance, they say, *"I'd like to speak to the voice of desire."*

3. The facilitator asks, *"Who am I speaking to?"*

4. The person or group being facilitated responds, *"The voice of desire."*

5. Speaking as the voice being spoken to—as desire—the facilitator through that voice asks a series of questions of that voice, hearing from those being facilitated what insights and gifts that voice brings into the life of the self and others.

6. When the first pole has been fully given voice, the facilitator speaks to the other pole in the same manner.

7. There is then an exploration of the relationship between the poles that helps reveal the health and maturity in that relationship.

8. The facilitator then asks to speak to a perspective – a place of still awareness - that transcends yet includes both poles, to explore whether anything in addition can be witnessed from that perspective that was not previously elicited from the perspective of the individual poles.

9. The facilitator then invites the Still Point or Virtue of Being of that polarity to come forward, which brings those polar dynamics to stillness. This is a profound, transcendent experience for most people. There is less verbalization here and the facilitator asks questions more along the line of "what does this feel like," which for every Still Point is virtually always an experience of deep Peace outside of space and time, together with other interesting spiritual and/or egoless qualities related to that bandwidth of ourselves. Before the first experience of a particular Still Point, many people have never experienced that quality of transcendence, and yet there is a realization that it has always been present and available, and they will often acknowledge as much. Sometimes that Still Point is not accessible for a person,

and being in a group listening to that Still Point voice speak up through others sometimes creates an opening for that person to access what is already there that has been hidden.

10. From there, the facilitator speaks to the transcendent Virtues of Becoming and Doing—the Character Virtues—that flow from the Virtue of Being, and the transcendent Polar Virtues that arise out of the Virtue of Doing. Each of them is asked to express the profound Healing, Flourishing, and Spiritual gifts that they offer the self and others. Again, those being facilitated are sharing this transcendent Wisdom, which has been pre-existing from within themselves.

There are of course all sorts of variations on the theme when facilitating. When this voice-dialogue approach is pursued on a one-on-one rather than a group basis there is an opportunity for a great deal of individual exploration.

Even as the IPP polarities and virtues are universal and archetypal, each individual tends to give them voice in a way that provides a somewhat different perspective or expression than another person would, which gives everyone in an IPP voice-dialogue group facilitation a powerful opportunity to open themselves up to many new insights regarding how the same aspect can manifest and share its gifts. Even as we may not stably embody the Virtues immediately, each time after we have spoken from, as, and to them, and enacted them, we reinforce them in our lives—such as virtues arising from the Intent Polarity of Abundance, Gratitude, and Generosity. In this way, authentically experiencing such transcendent qualities through voice dialogue is a powerfully reinforcing touchstone for personal practice that can be remarkably impactful.

An IPP facilitator is also trained to work with meditative and other facilitative techniques. Those who practice IPP over time learn to self-facilitate and to do inner work, and move in the world naturally and organically through the resonances and harmonies of the IPP polar and virtue ecosystem.

Another important aspect of IPP that becomes salient through facilitation of polarities is how we can awaken and interconnect multiple fragments within ourselves. For instance, when we speak from the voice of aversion, in addition to aversion being aware of its primary function of pulling away from something, we find that aversion is often more aware than the conscious self of reasons that the self has an aversion to a particular thing, and can identify additional aspects within the self that are relevant to the related issue. This can be a profound revelation of uncovering and self-discovery. This process helps us heal, makes us more whole, and enables us to flourish more fully.

In addition, by speaking to or from polar aspects in voice dialogue, we can better discern their level of maturity. For instance, as previously suggested, if we find that desire and aversion are generally in deep conflict, it follows that they are not very mature. We in turn learn to develop greater maturity in this regard. Similarly, if a polar voice cannot be found, it is stunted and/or has been repressed. It can usually be awakened fairly easily through the work of an IPP facilitator, who is trained to explore with those being facilitated the relationship of the poles on the trajectory of maturity on the way to interpenetration and then Unity. It is helpful to discover the level of functionality and maturity in every dimension of ourselves. Just being aware of the maturity trajectory and where one is on that maturity spectrum regarding that aspect of ourselves is an attractor to growth, integration, and free-flowing functionality.

To complete an overview of what appears in every Primary Polarity chart, the following is a brief description of three additional aspects that you can note on the Intent Polarity chart, which adds nuance to IPP practice:

- First, if access to either of the poles of a polarity or to any of the three Virtues is blocked, there is a word on the chart representing a pathology that tends to result. For instance, if you are blocked from the Still Point of Satisfaction, Contentment, Fullness, and Abundance in the Intent Polarity, you tend to come from a place of chronic deficit in attitude and outlook, which is the case for most people prior to IPP training.

- Second, just beneath the title on the Intent Polarity chart is a polar activator: dissatisfaction/inspiration. These are two related polar qualities that tend to trigger the polar dynamics of this particular polarity. When you are dissatisfied or inspired, the desire/aversion dynamic activates. The polar nature of the polar activator enables it to integrate into its own Unity as a part of IPP practice.

- Third, at the bottom of the chart the fully realized and integrated polar dynamic is designated as providing the "Gift of Sacred Intent." Every IPP polarity is given a "Sacred" designation to emphasize that every aspect of our humanity in its Fullness has a sacred dimension to it, each contributing in multiple interconnected ways to the flourishing of our Sacred Humanity. To the extent that a polar dimension is fully functioning with virtues stabilized as described here, it is flourishing, and we become more aware of and manifest its Sacred nature. In this context we also become more aware of the Sacredness of all our relationships and our intimate interconnections with all life and manifestation, as well as the importance of Loving Stewardship for all Creation.

Deeper IPP Patterns, Structures and Practices

Many people experience significant individual and collective flourishing deriving from IPP as a spiritual, life, or organizational practice, without delving into the deeper IPP patterns, structures, and practices. However, understanding and working with those patterns, structures, and practices enables you to optimize your own flourishing and more fully contribute to the flourishing of others. Some of these patterns and practices will be briefly summarized in the following few pages before reviewing four additional polarities and how they support flourishing. Nevertheless, this information is not necessary to understand and appreciate the remainder of the book. If the content seems too dense or not personally relevant, please feel free to skip the remainder of this section.

It is helpful to understand the notions of "concrete," "subtle," and "causal" as we use them. These terms, derived from the Vedantic tradition, are used broadly in many awareness and meditative traditions, and I settled into using them early on in the development and practice of IPP. In the Vedantic tradition, *concrete* refers to the physical world, *subtle* refers to the world of thoughts and feelings, and *causal* refers to the still source—the *cause*—of thoughts, feelings, and the physical dimension. These three terms can also be understood more broadly as any spectrum of three degrees of refinement, where for instance one quality is more solid (concrete), the middle quality is more flowing and flexible (subtle), and on the other end is more refined and still (causal). These terms are referred to here with this broader sensibility. They represent a core three-part harmonic that is found in multiple dimensions throughout IPP and are summarized more fully in the notes.[11]

In terms of the qualities of every IPP polarity, the poles represent the "concreteness" of the consciousness and energy of the polarity. The flow of consciousness and energy between the poles is the subtle quality of the polarity, and that flow constitutes the "subtle field" of the polarity. The "causal" dimension of a polarity is the "transcend and include" position at the top of the polarity where integration is complete and the causal stillness of awareness resides. Yet there is an active witnessing quality, where there is a separation between the witnessing position and what is being witnessed.

When one drops into the still center, the Still Point, this is a quality of Non-Duality, where no separation of any kind exists. There are three qualities of the Non-Dual Still Point. For instance, as previously noted in the Intent Polarity, when we bring our more concrete and physical desires and aversions to stillness, the Still Point quality is "Satisfaction." When we bring the desires and aversions of our more subtle emotions and minds to stillness, the Still Point Quality is "Contentment." The deepest stillness arising from our most refined and spiritual or causal sensibilities is "Fullness." So, the three qualities of each Still Point reflect the manifestations of the Non-Dual Still Point of any IPP polar dynamic of the physical (concrete), mental and emotional (subtle,) and more pure spiritual awareness (causal) bandwidths of our humanity.

As noted earlier, sometimes for simplicity we use one term for all three qualities of a Still Point of a particular polarity, which summarizes the essence of all three levels of the Still Point. For instance, for the Intent Polarity, we often use as a summary designation of the Still Point of desire/aversion the word "Abundance." In addition, we sometimes refer to an actionable quality that arises from such a Still Point. For example, we often refer to a sense of profound Possibility that arises from being deeply centered in Abundance.

The "Light," "Love," and "Life" that flow through every Still Point are transcendent manifestations of the same three-part harmonic: Light is the transcendent causal, Love is the Transcendent subtle, and Life is the transcendent concrete. As will be discussed, I will build on this core three-part harmonic to identify a five-part IPP Harmonic that resonates throughout IPP.

As appears in the Intent polarity chart and in every other IPP polarity chart on the following page, you will note that there is a shaded Fullness side of the Still Point, which represents the poles having moved beyond integration and become "not two"—a first step of Non-Duality—and an unshaded emptiness side of the Still Point, which represents a quality of awareness without an object, an empty awareness, which naturally arises on the other side of that Fullness.

These Full/Empty qualities of each Still Point form their own polarity; they are full and empty qualities of the same causal Stillness. The empty side is always the same—just emptiness. There is almost always a sense of profound Peacefulness and of being outside of space or time.

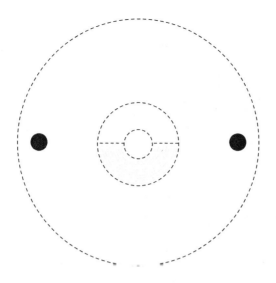

(The empty/full polarity is a causal variation of the subtle polarity, interior/exterior, and the concrete polarity, inside/outside.)

As one practices with this Still Point polarity there are the identical progressions of maturity towards integration and maturity as found in any polarity. At the Still Center of any Primary Polarity, over time one begins to sense Fullness in the Emptiness and Emptiness in the Fullness (interpenetration), and that ultimately that they are Not Two. This is a second progression in Non-Dual attainment in IPP. This second quality of Non-Duality can be facilitated in virtually anyone by an IPP master facilitator, but stabilizing in this attainment usually takes years of practice. When experiencing this quality of Non-Duality regarding any Still Point, there tends to be a shift from where you experience the Light, Love, and Life. Rather than feeling them flow from a deeper Source through a "Still Point Portal," you come to perceive this flow arising from no discernable separate Source. There is merely a Non-Dual Source (as Ground), Light, Love, Life, and their Integrated Expression. Another variation on a transcendent expression of the IPP harmonic is: One, Light, Love, Life, Whole, which is discussed in Part 2.

When you stabilize in the second Non-Dual quality of the Still Point of a polarity, you experience that there is a flow from this Non-Dual Ground to the causal stillness, then to the subtle flow in the polar field, on to the concreteness of the polarities, and finally to the integrated expression of all of these harmonic qualities. This amounts to a five-step progression of "Ground, causal, subtle, concrete, integration," which is a variation of a full five-part "IPP Harmonic" that shows up in many variations in IPP practice, and which makes IPP ultimately an aesthetic practice. This is a descending or "involutionary" flow from a prior Unity (Non-Duality) to a multiplicity. You can also feel this IPP Harmonic flowing in the opposite direction, where the integrative experience becomes transmuted into the Ground, and the Ground becomes the integrative experience: Ground, concrete, subtle, causal, Integration. This is an ascending or "evolutionary" flow from a multiplicity to a Unity. This two-way flow is a manifestation of the Foundational Creation Polarity of descending (involution)/ascending (evolution), a "meta-polarity" in IPP practice that is briefly addressed later in this section. In its deepest manifestation you will experience that the Source of Ground or Integration has the same quality of Non-Duality. The three core "notes" of the IPP Harmonic are framed by two transcendent qualities represented by capitalized words as follows: Ground, concrete, subtle, causal, Integration—or reverse order of the core notes.

A third Non-Dual practice in the context of every polarity is to observe from your deepest place of witnessing awareness how you are experiencing a particular polar dynamic, which is also its own polarity: witnessing/witnessed. (witnessing/witnessed is a causal variation of the subtle polarity of individual/collective, and the concrete polarity of self/ other). When you work with this polarity, sometimes you will witness yourself concretely in this regard. Over time, through a more refined sensibility, you may witness the more subtle field of your consciousness and energies, and/or the consciousness and energies of a collective of which you are a part in that moment. A more advanced attainment is to experience this witnessing dynamic becoming universalized, so to speak, and there is a witnessing of Kosmic qualities.

Whatever variation on the theme that you experience, the practice is then to allow the witnessing quality to collapse into what is witnessed. In this practice you are essentially practicing the courage to die, so that you can experience what new manifestation of identity might then be re-born. This puts you on a trajectory of growth, maturity, and transformation in terms of ego identity and related dynamics.

Regarding the overall IPP structure or ecosystem, the Intent Polarity is the integrative capstone of the nine Primal Polarities that we are all born with. Note Schedule 1, the summary Primal Polarity chart. The nine Primal Polarities are foundational to the emerging Human World. As we mature and grow up, we tend to reach "further and further down" to consciously encounter and ideally embrace all the Primal Polarities as they already resonate unconsciously within us. The Intent Polarity is also the integrative capstone stage of the top four of the Primal Polarities—the Life, Perception, Awareness, and Intent Polarities— which compose the "Life World" or "Life Tier." The Life World or Tier, comprising these four stages, acts as the ground for the Human World, which arises out of it. The Human World is composed of the Concrete, Subtle, and Causal Tiers, each made up of four stages of human development. There is also a projected Non-Dual Tier of four stages beyond the Human World, which is an Integrated Tier in relation to the Human World Tiers. In summary, there are Ground, Concrete, Subtle, Causal, and Integrated (Non-Dual) Tiers of the Human World in an ascending order and Ground (former Integrated), Causal, Subtle, Concrete, and Integrated (former Ground) Tiers in a descending order.

The Intent Polarity itself is also the ground polarity of the first Concrete Tier of the Human World, which includes concrete, subtle, causal, and integrative polar stages (so characterized for purposes of explicating the IPP Harmonic in every Human World Tier, in addition to their other designated names). There is an identical IPP Harmonic in all the Human World Tiers, where the integrative stage of the prior tier acts as the ground stage and "gives birth" to the next tier of four stages each.

Immediately below the four stages of the Life World among the Primal Polarities is the single polarity that represents the Material World, the manifestation polarity (energy (wave)/mass (particle)).[12] Only as people reach significant maturity in their development is there a natural tendency to reach this far down to become fully conscious of and to directly experience these material world dynamics and related Virtues. The Material World Polarity will not be reviewed in this introduction to IPP.

The bottom remaining four of the nine Primal Polarities are the Foundational IPP Polarities. If you do not include the Foundational Polarities, IPP as a practice is complementary to virtually any philosophical or spiritual tradition in service of flourishing. When the Foundational Polarities are integrated into IPP practice there may be elements related to the Foundational Polarities that are not totally aligned with every person's beliefs, because they reflect assumptions relating to aspects of reality, divinity, creation, and identity. So as an IPP practitioner you can customize your practice by including or excluding any of the Foundational Polarities as you deem appropriate. On the other hand, we usually introduce Foundational Polarity practice as an experience to see how it resonates, but are flexible in training with regard to whether any Foundational Polarity is concerning. In any case, the Foundational Polarities provide IPP with a fullness of patterned integrity.

In descending order the Foundational Polarities are as follows:
1. The Reality Polarity (Consciousness/Spirit), which suggests a polar framing relating to ultimate Reality
2. The Divinity Polarity (Divine Feminine/Divine Masculine), which is a primary quality of the Divine within each of us and among all of us
3. The Creation Polarity (Ascending (Evolutionary)/Descending (Involutionary), which embraces the wholeness of the eternal process of Creation
4. The Identity Polarity (Universally Divine/uniquely personal), which helps each of us appreciate that the wholeness of our

identity comprises our oneness with the Divine (and the divine within all of us), showing up in our lives through expression of the gifts of the utter uniqueness of each of us

None of these Foundational Polarities is specifically addressed in this book, but each is illustrated at least once through a particular application in IPP practice.

The four Foundational Polarities are aligned Harmonically with the four post-polar stages of development in a Non-Dual Tier of development[13] beyond the Human World, as set forth in the Non-Dual—Foundational Polarity Overview Chart as Schedule 3. Note that the Foundational Polarities and Non-Dual Tier frame the Concrete, Subtle, and Causal Worlds as an expression of the IPP Harmonic. In an ascending or evolutionary direction of practice, the Foundational Polarities are the Ground, and the Non-Dual Tier is the Integration. In a descending or involutionary direction of practice the Non-Dual Tier is the Ground, and the Foundational polarities represent Integration.

The IPP Harmonic pervades IPP Practice. As an IPP practitioner, you can engage step by step into the fullness of the Harmonic. The multiple dimensions of the IPP Harmonic transcend our cognitive ability to keep track of them in the moment, even as they endlessly resonate in multi-dimensional ways through the jazz compositions of our lives. As you engage deeply in IPP practice, you learn to intuitively compose your life and relationships through the IPP Harmonic, even as you are already being composed by it.[14]

There is an advanced IPP practice that assumes Non-Dual attainment by the practitioner called the Descending or Involutionary Practice. It creates a framework for a practice oriented toward a passionate embrace of all life and manifestation explicitly through the IPP Harmonic. Note Schedule 4, the Non-Dual Involutionary Practice Chart. There is a corresponding Non-Dual evolutionary practice. Together they form a variation of the foundational IPP Creation Polarity: ascending (evolution)/descending (involution).

The Life Tier Polarities

We will now briefly explore the remaining three of the four Life Tier polarities in addition to the Intent Polarity, which has been the primary example for demonstrating the characteristics and practices related to all Primary Polarities. We share the four Life Tier polar dynamics in important ways with virtually all non-human living beings. They cover the territory central to most meditative traditions. Many people elect to begin IPP practice with a meditative emphasis, concentrating on the Life Tier polarities. Such a practice provides a strong foundation for Human World IPP practice. In recent years, many students have been introduced to IPP through one or more weeklong retreats, mostly meditative in nature, which emphasize working primarily with the Life Tier polarities.[15]

The four polarities in the Life Tier reflect the IPP harmonic, as do the four IPP polarities in each of the three tiers of human development. In ascending order the first stage of the Life Tier, the Life Polarity, is the most concrete stage of the Tier; the second stage, the Perception Polarity, is more subtle; the third, the Awareness Polarity, is more causal, and the fourth, the Intent Polarity, is the integrative stage of the Tier. The Material World Polarity just below the Life World polarities—the Manifestation Polarity—is the ground stage supporting the Life Tier. The foundational dynamics of life and consciousness arise through the Life Tier polarities. We will review these three Life Tier polarities in addition to the Intent Polarity in descending order.

Awareness Polarity (focus/open)

Just below the Intent Polarity is the awareness polarity. Whether you know it or not, you have access to a profound inner Stillness, which is the essence of being Awake in a transcendent sense. You are constantly engaged in the related polar dynamics—focus/open—when you are

Awareness

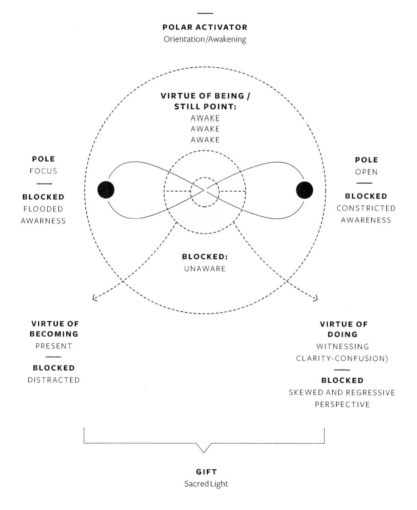

POLAR ACTIVATOR
Orientation/Awakening

**VIRTUE OF BEING /
STILL POINT:**
AWAKE
AWAKE
AWAKE

POLE
FOCUS

BLOCKED
FLOODED
AWARNESS

POLE
OPEN

BLOCKED
CONSTRICTED
AWARENESS

BLOCKED:
UNAWARE

**VIRTUE OF
BECOMING**
PRESENT

BLOCKED
DISTRACTED

**VIRTUE OF
DOING**
WITNESSING
CLARITY-CONFUSION)

BLOCKED
SKEWED AND REGRESSIVE
PERSPECTIVE

GIFT
Sacred Light

awake. They entail being open to what is arising in your awareness and focusing in that context. Most of us have an undisciplined awareness polar dynamic that tends to jump around a lot, whether we intend it to or not. Training and practice in disciplining this dynamic is central to a meditative practice and ultimately to optimal flourishing.

The Still Point of this polarity is the Stillness of Awareness, or being fully Awake. This Still Awareness is a deeper quality of yourself than your concrete physical senses or your subtle emotions or subtle thinking mind. You can be Awake in the moment and Witness (Virtue of Doing) your concrete sensory self and your subtle emotional and mental self and even your own ego. Eventually you can Witness your own awareness in the moment. Learning to function in life from this place of Stillness is life-changing. Learning to identify with this Stillness amounts to identifying with a deeper and more profound quality of who you already are. When you are Awake in this way you are by definition "Present," the Virtue of Becoming—"being in the moment." Fully stabilizing in this causal witnessing quality is not fully accessed in a structural way in terms of human development until one begins to inhabit the Causal Tier of human development, but this causal quality is always present, and one can transform one's life by practicing and stabilizing in this polarity.

Basic practices related to this Awareness Polarity would include the following:

- Practice your awareness being open, and practice being focused, and notice the inevitable focusing within the openness and openness within the focusing.
- Open your Awareness to and focus on some aspect of your concrete senses in the moment. For example, just touch your arm, and be aware that this touching brings you into the present moment, which can be extremely helpful when you have been distressed by something, for instance.
- Be aware of your emotions and thoughts. Over time you can cre-

ate a conscious gap between your Witnessing Awareness and your emotions and thoughts. The point is not to either repress or control them but rather to simply be aware of them in the moment as they arise without judgment. Paradoxically, when you create a conscious separation between your awareness and your emotions and thoughts, your emotions and thoughts no longer have control over you, even as you are not trying to control them. Witnessing in the moment our concrete senses and subtle qualities of emotion and mind represents the essence of classic mindfulness practice.

- Another framing of the prior practice description is to pay attention to what you are paying attention to. For instance, you may notice that you are being overly critical of yourself or others. Another example is that when you are grieving—which we all have occasion to do in our lives—you can pay attention to whether you are too immersed in dark or "what if" type thinking. By simply noticing such negativity or darkness, you can choose to redirect your thoughts and feelings for a bit to tend to your own wellbeing.

- Be aware of and witness the constructs conditioning your perception as set forth in the polarity chart for the Perception Polarity, and how they inevitably condition what you think you perceive.

- Be aware of your own ego. At first this is difficult to do in the moment. However, if on reflection you note when you have been triggered, for instance, or have behaved in a less than optimal way, you can reflect on that and over time learn to be more aware in the moment when you might be more egoic or reactive than is ideal. Your behavior over time will begin to evolve, influenced by the deeper Wisdom of simply being Awake.

- Another more advanced practice is being aware in the moment of your own awareness. (Note that this capacity does not normally arise until one's developmental center of gravity moves into the Causal Tier of Development.)

Perception Polarity (in/out)

Using our senses we perceive, taking in external or internal inputs through our concrete, subtle, and causal receptors, and we digest them through our concrete, subtle, and causal faculties, which results in a perceptual output, and is represented in the two polar qualities of "in" and "out." Note that the domain of perception is often conflated with the domain of awareness, but it is helpful to tease apart these dynamics even as they are inevitably interpenetrating.

Part of practicing with this polarity is to become familiar with the conditioning of our perception both in terms of input and output in ways that most of us do not normally become conscious of until the later stages of human development. This conditioning includes: you significantly construct what you perceive, which is in part related to your stage of development; your perceptions are also embedded in endless social and experiential contexts; you are likely unconsciously engaging in multiple projections and introjections with those around you.

Mastering being aware of and appreciating the impact of all these filtering dimensions of perception can take many years. However, simply learning to be aware of and present to these conditioning filters can be transformational even in the short term. Ultimately, you will come to see in the moment how extensively you construct and filter your perception. Only by bringing to awareness such pervasive conditioning can you paradoxically begin to see more clearly what is actually arising in the moment. As previously mentioned, qualities of witnessing and awareness in this regard involve the interpenetration with the Awareness Polarity.

The Still Point for this polarity, Openness, causes you to take a pause in the endless in/out feedback loops of Perception, and to be Open not only to a clearer sensibility of what is arising but also to sourc-

Perception

—

POLAR ACTIVATOR
Construction/Stimulus

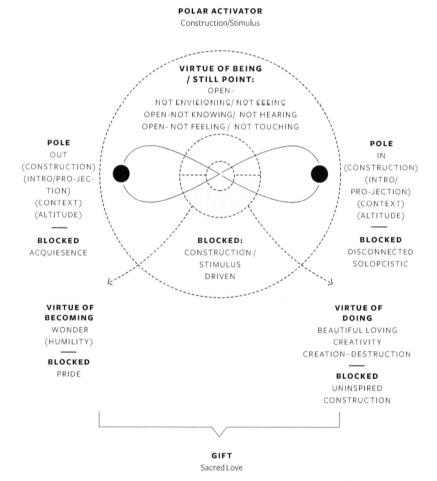

**VIRTUE OF BEING
/ STILL POINT:**
OPEN-
NOT ENVISIONING/ NOT SEEING
OPEN-NOT KNOWING/ NOT HEARING
OPEN- NOT FEELING / NOT TOUCHING

POLE
OUT
(CONSTRUCTION)
(INTRO/PRO-JEC-
TION)
(CONTEXT)
(ALTITUDE)

—

BLOCKED
ACQUIESENCE

POLE
IN
(CONSTRUCTION)
(INTRO/
PRO-JECTION)
(CONTEXT)
(ALTITUDE)

—

BLOCKED
DISCONNECTED
SOLOPCISTIC

BLOCKED:
CONSTRUCTION /
STIMULUS
DRIVEN

**VIRTUE OF
BECOMING**
WONDER
(HUMILITY)

—

BLOCKED
PRIDE

**VIRTUE OF
DOING**
BEAUTIFUL LOVING
CREATIVITY
CREATION- DESTRUCTION

—

BLOCKED
UNINSPIRED
CONSTRUCTION

GIFT
Sacred Love

ing a deeper Intuition and Creativity. Through this profound Openness you naturally develop a Virtue of Becoming, of Wonder at what can be Sourced deeper than the thinking mind, the feeling emotions, and visceral sensibilities. This also requires a profound Humility, whereby the ego self and the thinking mind must learn to be more Open to "not knowing." Another framing of this Virtue is becoming comfortable with "Not Knowing." By accessing a deeper connection to underlying Reality, and seeing more clearly the filters of perception, you become more deeply and authentically involved in the Doing Virtue of generating Beautiful, Loving Creativity. Since this is the subtle stage of this Life Tier, Love is always present when the transcendent is accessed.

The following are basic practices related to this polarity:

- Practice every day opening yourself to Wonder and Awe, to that which is beyond yourself and the constructs of your mind. For example, be open to the wonders of nature, even the beauty of one small flower bud. Always include having a sense of wonder and regarding the deeper Reality and Source, which is beyond the constructs of the subtle mind. A simple Wonder and Awe Practice can be profoundly healing, even transformational, and naturally generates a moment of pause and Openness. A Not Knowing practice is parallel to an Awe Practice.
- Pause the in-out cycle and be Open.
- The first transitional stage of Openness is to pause and make more considered choices rather than reacting automatically or habitually, with mental faculties subsumed in a cycling of constructs. This involves "meta-cognition," which most mature adults have access to.
- The second stage of Openness is to be more open to the primacy of Awareness and to be Intuitive in the moment. Like a martial arts fighter, if you are Present, you can react more quickly as well as Intuitively and Creatively, and be more "in the flow" than your thinking mind is able to be.

- The third stage is to be open to the Abundance that is there, and to which you may already have Opened yourself through practicing the Intent Polarity.
- The fourth stage of Openness is to be Open to the Emptiness in that Fullness, and the Light, Love, and Life that flows through that emptiness from the Source, which flows like "Living Waters."

Arising naturally out of Openness, the Virtue of Doing represents a conscious methodology of reframing arising from a deeper contact with the Source, which generates Beautiful, Loving Creativity—something that is more holistic and harmonious. The following progression can assist with this process: pause, deconstruct, intuit, reframe, and act. You can design personal, inter-relational, and organizational processes around this dynamic, as the Presencing Institute does, for instance, through applications of variations of "Theory U,"[16] a powerful approach using comparable insights being used globally to significant effect.

Life Polarity (expansion/contraction)

The expansion/contraction polar dynamics reflect the rhythmic and pulsating nature of all our primary physiological systems, which are most consciously accessible for many of us through our breathing. Following the breath is a foundation of most meditative practices. The Still Point of this polarity is coming to a state of physical Relaxation, being emotionally and mentally Calm, together with a deep spiritual Serenity or Tranquility. This gives rise to a profound Virtue of Becoming, of Acceptance, of not being in denial, of accepting "what is," even as we become clearer about what needs to be done in this moment. We will not access profound stability in this Still Point if we do not develop a deep disposition towards Transcendent Acceptance.

In this physiological bandwidth of yourself from a place of Accep-

Life

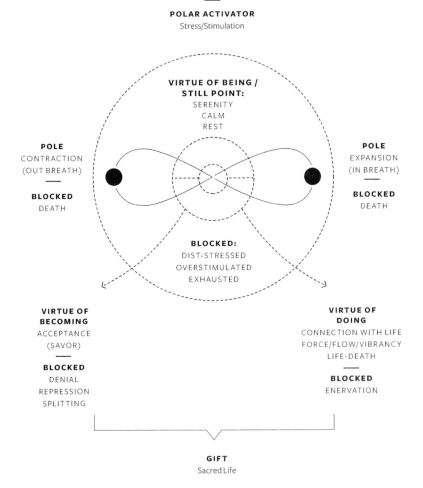

POLAR ACTIVATOR
Stress/Stimulation

**VIRTUE OF BEING /
STILL POINT:**
SERENITY
CALM
REST

POLE
CONTRACTION
(OUT BREATH)

BLOCKED
DEATH

POLE
EXPANSION
(IN BREATH)

BLOCKED
DEATH

BLOCKED:
DIST-STRESSED
OVERSTIMULATED
EXHAUSTED

**VIRTUE OF
BECOMING**
ACCEPTANCE
(SAVOR)

BLOCKED
DENIAL
REPRESSION
SPLITTING

**VIRTUE OF
DOING**
CONNECTION WITH LIFE
FORCE/FLOW/VIBRANCY
LIFE-DEATH

BLOCKED
ENERVATION

GIFT
Sacred Life

tance, Rest, Calm, and Serenity, you open the door to the Virtue of Doing, of connecting with the Vibrancy of the energy within yourself and all around you—of the Life Force. Getting well-grounded in these qualities of Stillness, Deep Acceptance, and profound Connectedness is a foundation for centering in Stillness through the full spectrum of your being—a primary goal of IPP. Most meditative traditions begin training in the context of this bandwidth, because stability and maturity here are such an important foundation for everything else that emerges through your humanity, while a lack of stability and maturity here destabilizes the rest of you.

Some basic practices:

- Settle into the three levels of the Still Point: Physical Relaxation (concrete), Mental and Emotional Calm (subtle), Deep Serenity and Tranquility (causal).
- Practice focusing on breathing, counting breaths until the mind wanders and then gently begin again. This practice can be frustrating until you let go of self-judgment, and you just accept the gradual way that your ability increases over time to become one with the deep physiological rhythm of your body. When you do this grounded in the Still Point you will feel a connection to the Life Force within yourself and beyond, which can yield an experience of the Divine Essence of all life. You also will be much more sensitive to the messages your body is sending you about its needs and wellbeing and sometimes even the wellbeing of life around you.
- With regard to this connection with the Life Force, begin to notice and then practice paying attention to the energetic vibrancy that is present in various settings. For instance, you can sense when there is low energy in a meeting and it feels stifling, and when there is high vibrancy, when everyone is participating and there is a sense of Abundance and Possibility.
- The two "yeses" related to Acceptance are to say "Yes" to What

Is—not being in denial of what is and being deeply Accepting of What Is. From this place of deep Acceptance and enhanced Clarity, say "Yes" again with Gratitude for your resulting Inspired Intent—what it is you want to do or not do in this moment and the next—given the reality of your circumstances.

Life Tier inspired meditation:

Following is a short meditation centering in the Still Point qualities of the Life Polarity, as well as all the other Life Tier polarities. This is a brief but powerful grounding practice, because Stillness in these most basic dimensions of yourself is a foundation for stabilizing the rest of yourself. Settle into your body with an erect posture and relaxed breathing. Allow your whole body to become relaxed. Bring forward within yourself these Still Point Qualities. You will notice below that all three Still Point Qualities of the Life Polarity are there, and only one quality related to the other Life Polarities. Pursue in the moment whatever variation of granularity works and is most helpful.

- Rest
- Calm
- Tranquility
- Open
- Awake
- Abundance

You begin to notice and then practice the related Virtues of Becoming alone or in tandem with these Still Point Qualities:

- Acceptance
- Wonder
- Presence
- Gratitude

The Virtues of Doing may not appear to be as naturally accessed in a pure meditative moment because they involve doing something, but you can do that silently and meditatively. Here's an example with the Life Polarity: when you are resting in Tranquility and Acceptance, in a state of deep Stillness, you may notice the Life Force more clearly than before, and that you are able to reach out and connect with the Life Force within you, within others, within all living things, within and through all manifestation.

In any case, all the Life Tier polar dynamics are pulsating constantly, and are and have always been embedded in your moment-to-moment life, but it is only through practice that you become more fully conscious of these Virtues and are able to center in Stillness and personally manifest and enact the Related Virtues.

Variations of practice in this arena are endless, and engaging in complementary meditative approaches can be enriching and helpful. Over time it is important to become fully conscious of and competent regarding all four of these Life Tier polar dynamics, and to manifest these Virtues as a part of everyday waking experience rather than accessing them solely through meditation.

The Relations Polarity (agency/communion) – the Polarity of Love

To initiate an IPP practice, many people start working with the Relations Polarity because it is the polarity of Love, in some ways the essence of flourishing. Overall, though, in order to engage the Relations Polarity for optimal flourishing, the Life World Polarities must also be reasonably functional and grounded in inner Stillness. Not only does each higher polarity ideally transcend, embrace, and transform the polarities beneath it, but more foundational polarities maintain their underpinning of higher-level awareness and functioning. This same top-down/bottom-up dynamic is relevant throughout human emergence, and having a practice that explicitly works with these patterns and polar dynamics is important for optimizing flourishing. This dynamic

Relations

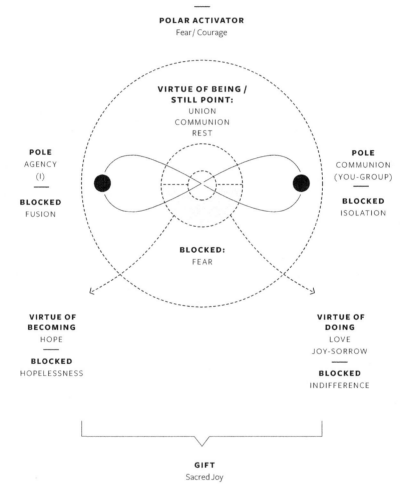

POLAR ACTIVATOR
Fear / Courage

**VIRTUE OF BEING /
STILL POINT:**
UNION
COMMUNION
REST

POLE
AGENCY
(I)

BLOCKED
FUSION

POLE
COMMUNION
(YOU-GROUP)

BLOCKED
ISOLATION

BLOCKED:
FEAR

**VIRTUE OF
BECOMING**
HOPE

BLOCKED
HOPELESSNESS

**VIRTUE OF
DOING**
LOVE
JOY-SORROW

BLOCKED
INDIFFERENCE

GIFT
Sacred Joy

is inherent in IPP practice through the ascending/descending Foundational Creation Polarity.

The Relations Polarity is the initial Human World polarity. It introduces the relational dimension of human experience, which is foundational for the rest of our lives. Since this relational dynamic arises in infancy, a concrete description of this polarity in our infancy or childhood would more appropriately be "me/you" or in our childhood and adolescence another concrete variation of "me/group." In our infancy and as toddlers we are only aware of one of the poles: ME. However, for the purpose of practicing with adults, that concrete polarity has been given a subtle polarity framing of agency/communion. (There is a subtle and causal variation of every concrete polarity.)

Among other things, "Agency" represents the qualities of choice and of conscience. "Communion" represents the polar quality of being in relationship, of connecting and communing, in contrast to any sense of separation. Primary dimensions of relationship include being in relationship with self, others, and collectives such as family, organizations, and community at all scales, as well as being in relationship with all life, all manifestation, and with the Transcendent or Divine. While physical relationships represent more concrete qualities of relationship, there are also more subtle qualities, such as being in relationship through shared assumptions, values, concepts, and agreements. We can also sense that we are all connected through a shared oneness of Spirit and Being. The bottom line is that people are relational beings in both the most basic and the most elevated ways.

Through facilitation and practice, you work with this polarity in the same manner as with every Primary IPP polarity. The least developed experience of the polarity is when you experience the poles of agency and communion as opposites with a strong preference for one pole or the other. The next step of maturity involves an ability to easily hold either pole, but only one at a time. That can further develop into being able to hold both poles simultaneously, beginning to experience a mutually complementary relationship between them, where you become conscious of the deep reciprocity dynamics that happen in every relational context. Then, you can begin to experience the poles as interpenetrating—an experience of "agency-in-communion" and "communion-in-agency." One implication of the latter is that your sense of meaning becomes deeply connected to a sense of purpose greater than yourself. One implication of the former is that in a collective, you become aware of how important it is to tend to the conscience and concerns of every member. Each step in this progression represents an advance toward developing maturity in a relational context. Each step is measurable and can be correlated with specific stages of human development. Hence, being aware of and working with this progression in this polarity is an attractor to personal growth and developing maturity in all categories of relationship.

The Still Point of agency/communion is an experience of Trust. This is ultimate Trust in something Transcendent, however you frame that, such as Trust in the Ultimate, God, Spirit, Absolute, Higher Self, etc. Trust is a concrete third-person quality of Stillness for this polarity. A more subtle second-person quality of Still Point is to Commune with the Transcendent. A more causal first-person manifestation of the Still Point is Union. These qualities of the Still Point are initially meditative, and over time can be stabilized and brought into one's moment-to-moment daily experience. For ease of reference here, this Still Point Virtue of Being will be referred to simply as Trust.

Because fear is normally present in any relational environment (the polar activator along with courage), you might say that the "job" of fear is to protect the self from dangers that might arise in any relational environment. Because we spend our lives constantly negotiating what to trust and what not to trust, what to fear and what not to fear, accessing and stabilizing in this Still Point is particularly challenging for many people. Yet paradoxically by being stably centered in Trust, you can be more present, and clearer and wiser about who and what to trust and not trust, and to what degree.

This Still Point generates an attitude of Hope as the Virtue of Becoming. This is not an everyday hope for specific things, but rather a deep dispositional Hopefulness. It includes an inner assurance that whatever arises can be dealt with wisely and well, which can be an enormous gift to the self and others. In this way, for example, you might be the one who is helpful and uplifting to others around you, even if you are the one who has suffered a loss or is experiencing a disability—or is even dying. When Trust is deeply inhabited and Hope is present, the dominant quality that flows through a person as the Virtue of Doing is unqualified and unlimited Love. This quality of Love and the related transcendent qualities of Empathy and Compassion are not limited to humanity, but extend also to the entire Life World, to this planet and to the entire Kosmos.

This polar dynamic demonstrates that it is no coincidence that variations of these three Virtues are clustered together so frequently, such as in Faith, Hope, and Charity. It is also no surprise that even a partial expression of such Love is encountered in most of our lives so infrequently outside of our closest family and friend relations (if even there), given the human proclivity to allow egoic qualities and fears to remain so central in our lives. However, IPP provides a practice framework for working with and growing into these Transcendent qualities, including opening a channel for transcendent Love and its related qualities to flow through us. It is a lifelong project to fully inhabit and enact the Virtues associated with the Primary Polarities, such as Love, but one great gift of IPP is that we can fully access and experience them in practice. They are simply there within us. Because Love is the very essence of flourishing, there is no more important Virtue to practice.

One of the Foundational Polarities, Divine Feminine/Divine Masculine can be utilized particularly powerfully when working with Love as the Virtue of Doing. In voice-dialogue facilitation of the Virtue of Love, the facilitator asks to speak to the Masculine or Yang voice of Love and explores the gifts of that Transcendent quality of Love. The Feminine or Yin voice of Love is then engaged in the same conversation. Next to be explored is the voice of Love with Feminine and Masculine qualities integrated. Quite often people find that they have a powerful sense of either the Masculine or Feminine qualities, but not both, let alone the richness of combining them both. You learn in multiple ways that whatever your gender orientation, fully embracing the transcendent qualities of both enriches and deepens your primary orientation, even as you are better empowered through this practice in the moment to apply the gifts of either as needed.

The Polar Virtues which arise out of Love—Joy/Sorrow—are particularly powerful. When you are facilitated into Sorrow, you experience a profound empathetic embrace of all suffering without limit. You have the inner Stillness and Presence to be able to behave appropriately and Lovingly and Compassionately in any circumstance—say, for instance, in a scene of genocidal carnage, where one does what is possible to comfort and assist others beyond any normal human capacity. (Note that this quality of Sorrow is in essence shorthand for passive empathy and active compassion.) It is just as startling to access Joy, because you can sense immediately that Joy is not fully accessible without accessing Sorrow, as they both arise out of Love. This is perhaps the greatest paradox of all, in that the messages that tend to come from the world we live in would have us avoid sorrow to access joy, and yet only by descending below all things in profound Empathy and Compassion do we rise above all things in the quintessence of human flourishing, by experiencing Joy/Sorrow grounded in Love, Sourced through Trust, and buoyed up by Hope.

There is significant research supporting the proposition that the Relations Polarity is a primary doorway to the essence of flourishing. Several research studies concluded that five elements of the Relations Polarity yield the highest leverage principles supporting human resilience and flourishing.[17] Those five principles are as follows:

- Being in a more deeply connected and vibrant relationship with one's higher and wiser self, with other people, with one's Source of spiritual wisdom, with the earth and its creatures, and with the kosmos (communion).

- Having an "internal locus of control" while maintaining the capacity of choice and being true to the integrity of one's deepest wisdom and values, regardless of circumstances (agency).
- Having a sense of purpose and meaning based on contribution to the greater good (i.e., communion-in-agency when these two poles interpenetrate).
- Having a profound sense of hopefulness, not in terms of hoping for specific outcomes (attachment), but rather having an attitude of being able to respond to whatever arises in each moment with wisdom, integrity, compassion, and courage. (This is known as transcendent Hope.)
- Having a deep experience of Love, the Virtue that penetrates and lubricates all these other virtues. Love, empathy, and compassion, both for self and others, are at the very heart of much research for creating personal, family, and community Flourishing (Love).

The Relations Polarity does not just provide a list of principles to optimize; it provides a profound understanding of how they interrelate and support one another in an ecosystemic context grounded in Love. Working well with these principles not only creates wellbeing (physical, emotional, mental, and spiritual), but is also proven to robustly improve stress resilience, human happiness, and self-actualization, which are all goals of individual and collective flourishing.

Trust, the Being Virtue in the Relations Polarity, into which the poles collapse and out of which the other Virtues flow, is missing from this list of research-based high-leverage flourishing principles. If Love is the primary lubricant of flourishing, Trust is the state of Beingness that is open to the Source out of which this unlimited and unqualified Love flows. Most research misses the spiritual qualities of Beingness, although spirituality as such is increasingly being recognized as an essential element of flourishing. The Sacred Stillness of the Still Point can and should be the conscious center of one's Being even as all manifestation is imbued with the Divine. This is why on each Primarily Polarity chart there is a designated shorthand sacred summary gift. In this instance, the Relations Polarity is designated the Polarity that represents the gift of Sacred Joy.

One powerful approach for beginning an IPP practice is to focus on the polar dynamics and Virtues related to the Intent Polarity, together with those of the Relations Polarity. Consider the interpenetrating power of the respective Virtues of these two polarities: Hope and Gratitude, Love and Generosity, all grounded in Trust, Abundance, and Possibility. The collective polar high-functioning and realization of the Virtues of these two polarities will in turn be reinforced by the healthy polar functioning and realized Virtues of all the other Life Tier Polarities and ultimately all the Primal Polarities.

The Virtue of Doing of the Relations polarity—Love—plays a central role in the primary Meta-Harmonic of IPP Practice. *Love* as the most involutionary Virtue of Doing of the entire Human World is a subtle quality. The most involutionary and concrete Virtue of Doing of the concrete Life World Is *Life* (vibrantly connecting to the Life Force). Unique Compassionate Embrace from the Identity Polarity is the most involutionary Virtue of Doing of the Foundational Polarities, which are the most involutionary set of polarities of all the Primary Polarities. Through the full Spectrum of the Primary Polarities, these comprise the most dominant and archetypal subtle (Love), concrete (Life), and integration (Unique Compassionate Embrace) Virtues of Doing of the Primary Polarities.

To complete the full Harmonic (adding "ground" and "causal" to subtle, concrete, and integration), the most involutionary stage of the Unified Tier acts as the Ground. The ultimate stage of the Causal Tier of the Causal Human World has causal "Light" as its Virtue of Doing. This particular Harmonic progression of Ground, Light, Love, Life, and Unique Compassionate Embrace constitutes "the" involutionary Meta-Harmonic of the Primary Polarities, which represents the full developmental spectrum of humanity. Love is at the essential center of the five-part harmonic progression, whether one is moving in an involutionary or evolutionary direction.

To further emphasize the overwhelming importance of Love, let us take a closer look at an aspect of the Identity Polarity (uniquely personal/Universal Divine). The Polar Virtues that emanate from the Virtue of Doing, Unique Compassionate Embrace are Freedom/Love. These Polar Virtues emphasize the centrality of Love as an ultimate integrative expression of the fully integrated Harmonic. Embracing someone with Love might seem to imply engulfing or constraining them, but paradoxically this most embracing of all Divine principles can only exist in tandem with Absolute Freedom. You can only Love in a Transcendent manner without restraint or reservation in a way that completely Liberates the Beloved. And you can be ultimately and transcendently Free only through the transcendent embrace of Love, which we all experience if we will but Awaken and embrace that Beauty.

In summary, IPP is designed to support you in more fully realizing your Identity as a Being of Light, Love, and Life who can engage in your own uniquely Divine compassionate embrace of all manifestation with Loving Inspiration and Creativity. In this way you can optimize flourishing both in your own life and in the life of others. This prepares us for Part 2: An Introduction to Integral Polarity Practice in Service of Leadership for Flourishing.

PART II

This Part 2 is an introduction to how IPP as a practice can be in service of leadership which generates interconnected individual, collective, and ecosystemic flourishing. I explain why we need mature leadership in the context of stages of human development to cope with the complex challenges of the twenty-first century and how IPP as a practice can over time support leaders in developing mature personal and leadership capacities.

I initially reference four of the nine Primal Polarities addressed more fully in Part 1 through the lens of leadership for flourishing and then explore the implications of that same lens for the first eight of the twelve additional polarities within the IPP ecosystem. Those twelve polarities are respectively aligned with twelve stages of human development of the Human World. The Human World is comprised of three tiers of development of four stages each. So, the eight IPP Human World polarities addressed in this Part 2 are aligned with the first eight stages of human development: the four stages in Concrete Tier of our childhood and the four stages in the Subtle Tier, which is the range of development of the large majority of adults in the developed world. The four stages of the Causal Tier, which perhaps less than one percent of adults inhabit, are not addressed in depth, but their powerful implications for leadership for a flourishing planet are introduced.

Life World Polarities

As noted in Part 1 the four Life World Polarities in ascending order are the Life Polarity (expansion/contraction), the Perception Polarity (in/out), the Awareness Polarity (open/focus) and the Intent Polarity (desire/aversion). Even though we are born with these four polar qualities relating to the basic dynamics of physiological functioning, perception, awareness, and intent, as we grow and develop, we ideally bring our highest awareness and capacities to inform and transform these dimensions within ourselves even as these transformed dynamics in turn remain powerfully foundational to the flourishing of each of us throughout our lives.

We will begin with a brief description of the relevance of virtues arising out of the four Life World Polarities as described in Part 1 related to one of many of their applications to leadership for flourishing, especially where there is a convening of a group that is experiencing deep differences over an issue ("Issue"). We call such convenings "Connecting Conversations."

Many other polar dynamics and related virtuous qualities are at play in such an arena (all of which would be worked with by an IPP trained leader-facilitator), but for illustrative purposes here, I will only reference the virtues related to the Life Tier polarities.

A leader who can personally manifest and share healthy IPP polar dynamics and related virtuous qualities with skillfulness for the leadership task at hand in service of flourishing is referred to as a "Flourishing Leader." A key point here is that the internal work we do also directly impacts our work in the world. The reverse is true as well. They are mutually informing.

When a Flourishing Leader is centered in the deep Calmness and Serenity of the Still Point of the Life Polarity, people tend to lean into that Stillness and Connect with that Leader as well as become more Present and Awake to what is arising in the moment. The Calm way a Flourishing Leader holds both the group and the Issue and Connects with them individually and collectively supports even participants who are experiencing trauma from their deep differences with others in the group in being more Open to exploring their previously unseen Connectedness to others in the group and beyond.

Creating awareness in a group of this Connectedness is typically facilitated in the following order:
1. Experience elements of their shared humanity (which are always fully present if rarely fully acknowledged);
2. Establish any agreements about facts and circumstances relat-

ing to the Issue (if any), together with Accepting that there are disagreements as to facts and circumstances (if that is the case - which it usually is when people come together with different cultural and political backgrounds), and that such disagreements are a reality is mutually Acceptable for this process;

3. Identify shared assumptions and values relating to the Issue (virtually always present albeit often inchoate to begin with);

4. Uncover any implicit agreements that are in place (if any) or that could be made based on their shared humanity, facts, assumptions, and values and make them explicit.

Through this process participants can experience and even savor the High Vibrancy that comes from a mutual realization and experience of such Connectedness.

When we say "Yes" to "What Is" in this regard by making both visible and felt shared Connections within or among groups where there has been deep disagreement, mutual distrust, perhaps even conflict, it is an extraordinarily Healing experience. From this place of Connectedness, a Flourishing Leader can facilitate a shared experience of Openness through which new Possibilities can emerge which often have not existed before in anyone's mind. With appropriate further facilitation a second "Yes" to moving forward together can often be discovered. By their very nature, such new Possibilities reflect qualities of Beautiful, Loving Creativity because they arise from a mutual exploration of the Participants' shared Witnessing of deeper and more holistic realities that transcend the mental constructs and biases which participants brought with them into the group facilitation. A shared sense of Wonder is often generated through a successful process in this regard, which lays the groundwork for further moving forward together.

It is particularly important that a Flourishing Leader holds and projects the virtuous qualities of the Intent Polarity well and deeply. The Intent Polarity is the fourth and highest emergent integrative capstone polarity of the four Life World polarities and by definition "transcends and includes" the qualities of the prior three polarities - and, for that matter, of all nine of the Primal Polarities. The Virtue of Being of the Intent Polarity is comprised of three transcendent qualities: being physically Satisfied, being mentally and emotionally Content, and being spiritually Full, which we refer to collectively as the transcendent quality of Abundance, which generates a related sense of Possibility.

There is significant precedent for the positive impact of an Abundant approach in communities. For many decades, a primary principle of community building has been the wisdom of coming from Abundance rather than scarcity[18]. A key point is that a Flourishing Leader is not just trying to encourage an attitude of Abundance, but rather models and can transmit a deep Beingness of Abundance. The latter is so much more powerful and effective in transforming any moment. When we focus on the Abundance of Possibilities that are available to generate a more fully flourishing community rather than dwelling on problems and deficits, we experience the profound High Vibrancy nature of that approach, and the results are transformative. The importance of this same quality of Abundance is relevant to every relational domain from families to large institutions and societies, and also yields a culture of deep Gratitude and profound Generosity (the related Character Virtues) which naturally flow from individuals and collectives experiencing Abundance. A Flourishing Leader who manifests and infuses into a group a profound transformative culture of Abundance and Possibility and who utilizes supportive institutional processes can be a remarkable catalyst for bridging divides of all sorts, generating strong collective agreements, achieving shared purposes, and engendering collective flourishing.

Human World Polarities

When it comes to introducing each of the following eight Human World polarities there is:

1. An initial brief description of the corresponding stage of human development at which that polarity first arises and how each of us tends to hold and work with that polarity as we grow into higher stages of development;

2. A description of how working with the polarity can support leadership for flourishing in a developmental context with an emphasis on one domain of leadership for illustrative purposes; and

3. In many cases a description of researched based approaches to leadership for flourishing in the body of the text or in the notes as an example of where IPP as a practice is aligned and could be of service as a practice.

Concrete Tier Polarities

In the IPP ecosystem there are four primary polar dynamics in the Human World which first arise in the "Concrete Tier" of human development, that is, during the concreteness of our childhood:

1. The Relations Polarity, which arises in our infancy, is the first and most foundational polarity in the Concrete Tier.

2. In ascending order, the "Power Polarity" then addresses the power dynamics which arise in every relational environment.

3. Following is the "Meaning Polarity," which has to do with integrating values and principles and a sense of meaning into our lives.

4. At the integrative fourth and final emergent stage of the Concrete Tier the "Purpose Polarity" arises, which involves the leadership polar dynamic itself.

With adult IPP practice we work primarily with more subtle or adult applications and versions of these four concrete polarities. For instance, a concrete version of the Relations Polarity which we deal with in child-hood would be me/other or me/group, but with adults we work primar-ily with a more subtle and flowing characterization of these qualities: agency/communion.

The Relations Polarity (agency/communion)

In Part 1, I emphasized how the practice of the Relations Polarity (RP) among other things generates unqualified and unlimited Love - the very essence of flourishing and the lubricant that connects and enhanc-es every other aspect of flourishing. A constellation of other particular-ly high leverage principles of resilience and flourishing comprising this polarity amount to the core ecosystem of flourishing grounded in Trust and Love, making RP the flourishing epicenter of the twenty-one polar dimensions of human awareness, function and flourishing that com-prise the entire IPP polarity ecosystem. As it naturally turns out, this same core ecosystem of flourishing comprises the foundational princi-ples and patterns of leadership for flourishing.

Because of its central importance to leadership for flourishing, I will describe the full polar dynamic of RP in this context. The IPP practice of RP highlights that people are profoundly relational beings in multiple dimensions of relationships such as with self, other, group, community, humanity, Nature, and Spirit. This is the "communion" di-mension of this polarity - a key principle of human flourishing. Agency, the other pole, represents that vital dimension of conscience and choice and having an internal "locus of control," which is an equally important principle of human flourishing. Variations of this polar dynamic are central to so many issues in society such as liberty and justice, individ-uality and community, rights and responsibilities, and the individual and the collective (the cultural emphasis of Western versus Eastern civ-ilizations). As with all IPP polarities, the trajectory of maturity of work-ing with this polarity moves from being embedded in and committed to one pole, to the flexibility of "either/or" choice, to the importance of holding them in a "both/and" manner, and then experiencing their integration. When the poles of RP are integrated, one deeply experiences a sense of "communion-in-agency" (which supports a sense of purpose in life greater than one's self) and of "agency-in-communion" (which for instance informs a Flourishing Leader in being aware of the importance of tending to the conscience, values, needs and creative input of each person in a group).

By bringing the relational dynamic of agency/communion to Stillness and thereby centering in the Stillness of a Transcendent Trust (Virtue of Being), we open ourselves to an attitude of profound Hope (Virtue of Becoming). From there, an unqualified and unlimited Love (Virtue of Doing) - the essence of flourishing - flows through us. As with all Virtues of Doing, there is a pair of transcendent virtues that flow out of Love: Sorrow (shorthand for profound Empathy and Compassion for the suffering of others and ourselves) and transcendent Joy (which co-arises with Sorrow).

As one example related to this polarity, RP patterns are central to the leadership represented in successful parenting. The following principles for optimal parenting consistent with RP patterns are derived from a comprehensive review of research relating to attachment theory[19]:

1. Provide your children safety and protection (Trust). This enables children to feel secure in venturing out, exploring, and knowing that they can return to the safety of their parents' embrace.

2. Be attuned to and empathize with the feelings and concerns of your children (Empathy). Listen to your children and help them feel understood and loved.

3. Soothe and comfort your children when they are hurt or in distress (Compassion). Be a source of unlimited and unqualified Compassion.

4. Express delight and Joy in your children's very existence (Joy).

Make them feel that that they are loved and celebrated without limitation or condition.

5. Support your children in developing their capacities consistent with their interests and creative inclinations rather than insisting that they pursue your preferences and expectations (Agency).

In summary, these principles provide a framework for supporting healthy patterns of attachment, growth, and development and more than anything else for Loving our children into Happiness, Wholeness and Flourishing.

More generally the RP patterns collectively provide a foundational framework for leadership and group flourishing, whether it is being a parent, a teacher, a leader of a private, civic, or public organization, etc. As with the patterns of all IPP polarities, these elements are not just a list of principles but rather patterns of consciousness, energy, and function which ecosystemically interrelate, mutually inform, and support one another. The following primary attributes of leadership in support of flourishing arising out of RP patterns are aligned with well researched principles of leadership[20] which can all be supported and enhanced in the context of practicing with RP and other related polarities:

1. Leadership begins with being personally trustworthy and sustaining an institutional framework and process for moving forward, which works well, that is, can be trusted to support outcomes for clearly defined purposes. The additional dimension for a Flourishing Leader trained in this polarity is that she is centered in a transcendent quality of Trust and profound inner Calm which also generates the transcendent qualities of Hope and Love. (Trust).

   a. Hold and nurture a container of trust in the group or organization, or broader society when a societal leader. This capacity is dramatically increased when a leader is deeply centered in transcendent Trust. Transcendent

Trust is a place of no fear, and a leader who embodies and shares this quality engenders greater trust in a collective. This is an example of an additional Virtue of Being that would complement the quality and success of Connecting Conversations which were described in the context of the Life World polarity virtues.

b. Support and sustain a culture of trust, which includes modeling and insisting upon mutual integrity, transparency, and trustworthiness.

c. From an environment of trust, courage should be expected to arise individually and collectively. Yet note that in IPP practice we discover that in a relative sense there is a healthy quality of fear that exists to protect from real danger and is in a polar dynamic with courage. In this context we uncover that healthy fear has a quality of courage embedded within it and healthy courage similarly carries a seed of fear's wisdom of not taking foolish risks.

2. A leader should Love those she leads including with Empathy and Compassion in a spirit of Joyfulness, expressed in a way that is appropriate in the given context (Love and Joy/Sorrow).

a. Model Loving Kindness in leadership as appropriately expressed and manifested in the setting and circumstances (Love).

b. Be empathetic and truly listen to (get to know) those you lead both regarding their own personal circumstances and appreciatively receive feedback relating to their experiences in the institutional context (Sorrow - passive Empathy). IPP training increases one's sense of developmental stages and related dynamics such as developmental modalities of expression, which can make a profound positive difference as to how effective one is in both listening and communicating empathetically. IPP training in working with developmental diversity is important for every leadership setting including for instance when facilitating Connecting Conversations.

c.   Be helpfully responsive in terms of personal issues and gratefully responsive regarding organizational feedback (Sorrow - active Compassion).

d.   Be appreciative of each person for whom you have stewardship even in the context of challenging circumstances, personal mistakes, etc. Take frequent opportunities to say thank you for a job well done and to celebrate frequently as a community (Joy).

3. A leader should honor peoples' agency including but not limited to the following (Agency):

a.   Honor each person's conscience and values (including your own) and encourage feedback in this regard rather than silence.

b.   Recognize and honor each person's strengths and take account of and adjust for weaknesses (including your own).

c.   Create opportunities for fostering personal stewardship and leadership as well as followership, and when appropriate be willing to follow the leadership of those you lead.

d.   Encourage and create opportunities for individual creativity to emerge and the fruits to be harvested and applied as appropriate.

e.   Encourage and create opportunities for personal development and growth in ways that align with people's interests and passions. This is also the domain of "exemplar leadership," the leader modeling the character-based transformation that she expects others to grow into.

    f.   Support deep synergy of these qualities of Agency and Communion integrating (communion-in-agency and agency-in-communion).

4. A leader should create and encourage qualities of communion including but not limited to the following (Communion):

    a.   Help develop social skills and emotional intelligence of those you lead along with leadership training which includes working with developmental diversity.

    b.   Work collaboratively and support strong teamwork.

    c.   Encourage and support a sense of community in the organization.

    d.   Encourage and create opportunities for collective creativity to emerge and the fruits to be harvested and applied as appropriate.

    e.   Encourage High Vibrancy relationships and utilize organizational design and processes which support and sustain High Vibrancy.

    f.   Encourage and create capacity for developing High Vibrancy not only within the group but with additional categories of relationship such as: self, other, community, Nature, and Spirit in an ecosystemic context.

    g.   Create deep synergy of these qualities of communion with qualities of agency. (Again: agency-in-communion and communion-in-agency)

5. A leader should engender a culture of Hope grounded in Trust and Love (Hope).

    a.   Hope in this transcendent sense is the confidence that we can deal well and lovingly with whatever arises.

    b.   Hope is also related to developing and supporting the important qualities of Perseverance and Grit in service of shared purpose.

    c.   This quality of Hope is deeply connected to the leader holding well the prior Intent Polarity by creating a sense of Abundance and Creative Possibility, and being Grateful and dealing Generously with the opportunities and challenges that arise.

6. A leader should help keep an orientation on fulfilling the purpose of a group in an expansive manner and inspiring the group in this regard (purpose in the context of agency-in-communion and communion-in-agency).

    a.   Align and connect individual assumptions to shared assumptions.

    b.   Align and connect individual values to shared values.

    c.   Align and connect shared values to collective agreements.

    d.   Align and connect collective agreements to the purpose of the group.

    e.   Note the spirit and expansive direction of such alignment and connection and further align and connect the purpose of the group to be of service to the greater good in an ecosystemic context.

All further descriptions of IPP polarities in support of leadership for flourishing build upon or are complementary to RP patterns and qualities of leadership in support of flourishing, which we refer to as "Foundational Patterns of Leadership for Flourishing." As noted, each successive emergent IPP polar dynamic transcends and includes the qualities and dynamics of all prior emerging polarities. That is the good news. IPP is a practice that enables us individually and collectively to work on more flourishing qualities of Being, Becoming and Doing through the full spectrum of our individual and collective humanity in an ecosystemic context. The challenging news is that less-than-optimal func-

Power

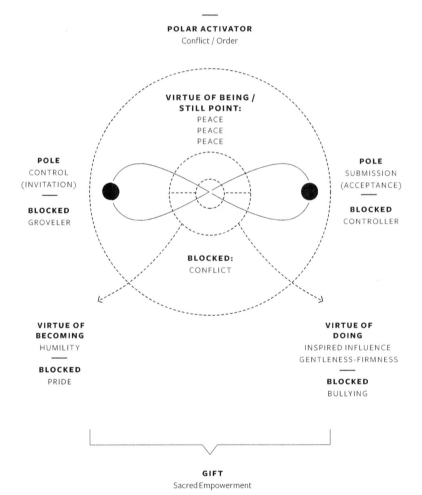

POLAR ACTIVATOR
Conflict / Order

**VIRTUE OF BEING /
STILL POINT:**
PEACE
PEACE
PEACE

POLE
CONTROL
(INVITATION)

BLOCKED
GROVELER

POLE
SUBMISSION
(ACCEPTANCE)

BLOCKED
CONTROLLER

BLOCKED:
CONFLICT

**VIRTUE OF
BECOMING**
HUMILITY

BLOCKED
PRIDE

**VIRTUE OF
DOING**
INSPIRED INFLUENCE
GENTLENESS-FIRMNESS

BLOCKED
BULLYING

GIFT
Sacred Empowerment

tionality of each prior polar dimension is suboptimizing to the whole and therefore calls for continual therapeutic or "shadow work" within the individual and the collective. IPP helps map and diagnose such pathologies individually and collectively and provides practices in support of transparency, integration, growth, and flourishing.

The Power Polarity (control/submission) (subtle version: invitation/acceptance)

Developmentally the Power Polarity first arises a half-step above the Relations Polarity. It brings structure into the relational domain. There are power realities in any relational environment, and everyone must learn how to work with this phenomenon. Even as the Relations Polarity first arises in infancy grounded initially in developing a sense of "me" in a passive way, the control pole of the Power Polarity enables the toddler to assert herself as a self with wants and needs. This is initially the mature stage of the toddler self-centric perspective, but naturally unfolds into working with the power realities of complex relational environments.

Our egos tend to be closely identified with the control pole. Yet as with all polarities, both poles - control and submission - are equally important qualities of power. Sometimes there is a tremendous power in submitting appropriately - for example, to submit to wise guidance, to a designated leader, to a set of values, to agreements, to the purpose of an organization of which you are a part, or to a spiritual path. And again, as with every polarity, this power dynamic is not just a tug of war between two opposing poles. In the trajectory of maturity, these polar qualities learn to cooperate and collaborate and ultimately begin to flow into one another, both being in service of one's core values, agreements, purposes, and deeper inspiration.

As with all polarities one ultimately experiences that there is a seed of submission within control, and control within submission. This is the essence of "servant leadership," a mature manifestation of leadership for flourishing. Servant leadership models leading by serving and learning and teaching that serving is leading. Servant leaders inspire others by their example, and those who follow servant leaders are drawn to power of what might seem to some at first as a paradox.

As we drop into the Still Point, where the poles are no longer two, no matter what contentious issues exist in your life, there is a concrete sense of no conflict, a mental and emotional quality of Peacefulness, and a profound Spiritual quality of Peace that transcends cognitive understanding (collectively transcendent Peace). We can learn to hold this quality of transcendent Peace even amid chaos and conflict. To fully and stably access transcendent Peace, we need to develop a transcendent Humility ("Virtue of Becoming"). When we are humble enough to move our egos aside and dwell in Peace, a quality of transcendent Inspired Influence ("Virtue of Doing") flows out of that because we are touching into and intuitively responding to the Source of Inspiration through the Still Point of transcendent Peace. These Character Virtues of Humility and Inspired Influence which flow out of power grounded in transcendent Peace are qualities that are the opposite of how power is typically wielded.

The transcendent polarity which arises out of Inspired Influence is a quality of transcendent Firmness and transcendent Gentleness. When one exercises Inspired Influence, it does not necessarily mean that you are always gentle, although transcendent Gentleness is always available. The most profound transcendent Firmness can be accessed to deal with situations as appropriately needed as guided by Inspired Influence. An example would be dealing with a situation where a predator is in the act of attacking someone who is vulnerable – even as an inspired insight in the moment may call on a quality of transcendent Gentleness to calm things down. Both transcendent qualities are present, available, and blended as needed in the service of our deepest inspired Wisdom and Compassion. Often through IPP practice, if a person's disposition is to be primarily firm, there tends to emerge in that person a quality of a

Meaning

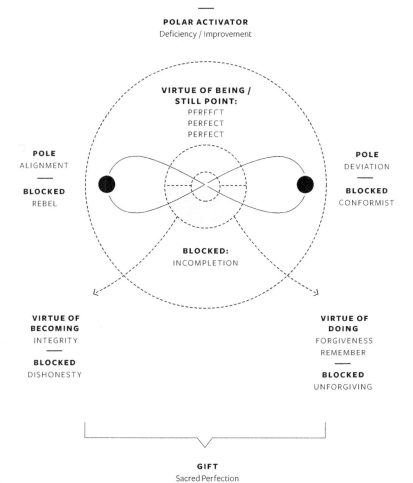

POLAR ACTIVATOR
Deficiency / Improvement

**VIRTUE OF BEING /
STILL POINT:**
PERFECT
PERFECT
PERFECT

POLE
ALIGNMENT

BLOCKED
REBEL

POLE
DEVIATION

BLOCKED
CONFORMIST

BLOCKED:
INCOMPLETION

**VIRTUE OF
BECOMING**
INTEGRITY

BLOCKED
DISHONESTY

**VIRTUE OF
DOING**
FORGIVENESS
REMEMBER

BLOCKED
UNFORGIVING

GIFT
Sacred Perfection

gentle firmness. Or if a person's primary disposition is to be gentle, that person often begins to exemplify a firm gentleness.

In a mature relational and leadership environment, a more subtle manifestation of control/submission tends to arise of "invitation/acceptance," even as more concrete manifestations of power and leadership are available as appropriate to the situation. In this version of the power dynamic the poles are already interpenetrating. Leaders are explicitly honoring the agency of followers (agency-in-communion), and followers are inherently acknowledging their own responsibility to the collective and shared purposes of the group (communion-in-agency). In this context mutual engagement often results in new emergent Possibilities. All of this is context dependent of course. For instance, often an order in a military chain of command simply must be promptly obeyed to avoid dire consequences. Nevertheless, practicing these invitation/ acceptance polar dynamics with mutual humility in appropriate situational contexts in an organization can increase opportunities for more Inspired and flourishing outcomes.

The Meaning Polarity (subtle version: alignment/deviation)

We conduct our lives in the context of our framework of meaning through discerning awareness. This is a capacity that is initially framed concretely, such as learning to follow rules or engaging in a repentance process in a Christian context. By around the age of eight most people can begin to engage competently with this polarity.

We normally do not work with this concrete version of the Meaning Polarity. A more subtle manifestation of the polar dynamic of meaning is alignment/deviation, which provides a more fluid and flexible quality of endlessly aligning or deviating regarding changing circumstances and growing awareness of and commitment to that which is most meaningful to us. On the other hand, if you are always coming from a place of feeling deeply flawed and endlessly adjusting in a spirit of "perfectionism," you can end up feeling "not enough" no matter how hard you try. This is a formula for endless frustration. When integrated into leadership such perfectionism will not only exhaust the leader in a group but everyone else as well.

As with any IPP polarity, if you are stuck in any pole or block out one of the poles you end up in a pathology. Are you driven to be a conformist? Do you identify as a rebel? IPP practice supports us in not fully identifying with any one pole, but rather for this polarity each polar quality learns to "to do its job" in tandem with the other pole with reference to our deepest framework of meaning.

When we drop into a place that brings that dynamic to a Still Point, there is no further need to align or deviate from anything. There is rather, an experience of transcendent Perfection in this Moment – being One with the Perfection of the Absolute, the Divine – however one frames that.

As with every Still Point, transcendent Perfection is initially a meditative experience in counterpart to the "relative" polar dynamic of alignment/deviation. But as with every polarity, as one matures in holding both the transcendent Stillness of the Still Point and the relative polar dynamic, they dance together and ultimately become "Not Two". As the leader comes from a place of the Abundance of transcendent Perfection, an effortless subtle flow of this alignment/deviation dynamic arises. The leader begins to deeply appreciate the opportunity to become more discriminating in every situation, and with no resistance to continuing to adjust with a deeper quality of transcendent Integrity (Virtue of Becoming). This is not an integrity aligned with our ego or concept of self but rather with the Wholeness and Perfection of every moment. When coming from such Abundance, course corrections are a part of endlessly exploring new creative Possibilities rather than struggling with endless insufficiencies.

From this place of transcendent Perfection and transcendent Integrity, we can see so much more clearly in our own lives and in the lives of everybody around us, that for the most part we are all just trying to do the best we can under the circumstances. "Life happens," and is inevitably full of challenges, missteps, and failures. We tend to become deeply and compassionately Forgiving (Virtue of Doing) of others - even of ourselves - for the shortcomings that we and others have and the suffering which we and others have caused. In an organizational environment, accountability is critical, but inspired leadership is always looking for opportunities for everyone to learn and grow from less-than-optimal performance and outcomes.

This does not mean that we are not responsible for injuries or damage that we may have caused or don't need to continue to work on our shortcomings, but from this place of transcendent Perfection, we can continue to work on the messiness of life and organizational challenges from a place of transcendent Integrity and transcendent Forgiveness. From transcendent Perfection we can see more clearly what needs to be done. And this is the paradox. Even as we can and should spend our lives course correcting - aligning and deviating - growing in Wisdom, Depth and Refinement, in a very real way we are always and already Perfect and Whole. Even if we make terrible mistakes or suffer terribly from the violations of others, we still rest in Perfection. We can continue on in a spirit of Acceptance, Gratitude, Love, Humility, and Integrity, always Forgiving in every moment.

Variations of Purpose Polarities

The fourth polarity that arises at the top of the four Concrete Tier stages is the Purpose Polarity (lead/follow). There is also a more subtle version of this same Purpose Polarity (facilitation/inquiry) which tends to arise at the top of the Subtle Tier. There is another polarity which independently arises at the top of the Subtle Tier, the Integrative Purpose Polarity (integration/re-integration). Since all these polarities are related to purpose – and "purpose" is so central to flourishing leadership

Purpose

—

POLAR ACTIVATOR
Meaninglessness / Searching

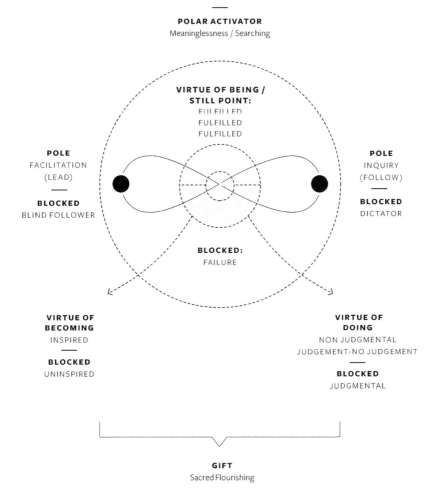

**VIRTUE OF BEING /
STILL POINT:**
FULFILLED
FULFILLED
FULFILLED

POLE
FACILITATION
(LEAD)
—
BLOCKED
BLIND FOLLOWER

POLE
INQUIRY
(FOLLOW)
—
BLOCKED
DICTATOR

BLOCKED:
FAILURE

**VIRTUE OF
BECOMING**
INSPIRED
—
BLOCKED
UNINSPIRED

**VIRTUE OF
DOING**
NON JUDGMENTAL
JUDGEMENT-NO JUDGEMENT
—
BLOCKED
JUDGMENTAL

GIFT
Sacred Flourishing

- they are grouped together as follows.

The IPP Purpose Polarity - (lead/follow) (facilitation/inquiry)

This IPP polarity, which reflects the dynamics specifically related to leadership, has two variations. The more concrete variation is "lead/follow." Most of us have access to this polarity before adulthood and continue to work with it for the rest of our lives. The more subtle version of that same IPP polar dynamic is "facilitation/inquiry." The lead/follow version will be addressed first.

This polarity initially arises at what we call the Mature Traditional stage of development, the top integrative stage of the Concrete Tier of development. In terms of authority those at Mature Traditional tend to look for a strong leader in an established hierarchy. They are group-centric in orientation and tend to be suspicious of those outside of the groups with which they identify, such as a faith, a race, or a political orientation. They tend not to be rigorous in terms of reasoning and are susceptible to narratives that are disconnected from reality, and which reinforce their worldview and validate their leader. One goal of Western educational systems is to support people in growing beyond the Concrete Tier of development including the capstone Mature Traditional stage, but a significant minority of adults never do. Population percentages in this regard have a lot to do with the fulfillment of basic life needs, and cultural and educational environments.

There are endless courses on leadership, but rarely does one find an offering on how to be a good follower. Yet as with every IPP polarity, one pole ("follow") is just as important as the other pole ("lead"). Having a bias against any pole is minimally immature and ultimately a pathology. Initially we identify solely with one pole: "I am a leader," or "I am a follower." This is the case for the most part for those both those at Mature Traditional and Early Modern stages. As a reminder we do not frame poles as nouns or sub-identities, but rather as functional aspects of a greater whole (lead/follow).

In the next step of maturity, in an "either/or" manner we chose or are chosen to enact one of the two poles: We are either leading or following. This is typical of the either/or roles that most of us have learned to take on at points in our lives or that our group or organization allot to us. Then we learn to hold both of those qualities at the same time. If you are a designated leader, you are conscious of the purpose you are following, and if applicable, those in a hierarchy that you in turn follow. In every moment you are also always listening, assessing the input of others even if you are an assigned leader, and ideally Open to following the wisdom and/or expertise that is available in the moment even as you maintain the stewardship of your assignment.

For instance, a soldier assigned to lead a platoon encounters a steep drop off, that all the members of the platoon will need to descend and is aware that one of the soldiers in the platoon is highly skilled at climbing and rappelling. In service of the purpose of the mission, that individual takes over leading the group by guiding everyone safely and efficiently down the steep incline. In turn as a designated follower, we are always ideally present to any circumstance where we might share some wisdom or be prepared to take on leadership. When roles are not so strictly designated - or at all - or when we are in the context of "mature" organizational and process models that are supportive of it, our leading and following qualities can both contribute as needed in the moment.

As we follow the maturity of the trajectory of these two poles, they flow into one another into a deeper Unity. We drop into the Still Point that brings the dynamics of this polarity to Stillness. That Stillness is present when we experience a quality of transcendent Fulfillment. From this place there is no further purpose to fulfill, towards which to follow, or to lead others. From an Absolute perspective this is always true: there is only Fulfillment. Recall that an experience of transcendent Fullness or Abundance is the Still Point of the Intent Polarity (desire/aversion), which is the polarity at the top integrative stage of the

Life Tier just as this Purpose Polarity is at the top integrative stage of the Concrete Tier. As a tier upshift, these two Still points of transcendent Fullness and transcendent Fulfillment are particularly resonant and reinforcing. So, for instance the place of transcendent Fulfillment is also a place of Fullness, Abundance, and endless Possibilities.

Coming from a place of transcendent Fulfillment we tend to be better able to exercise a transcendent quality of judgment in service of shared purpose without being judgmental of others, that is being transcendently Non-Judgmental (Virtue of Doing). For instance, from this Stillness we tend to be able to see so much more clearly whether we are aligned with shared assumptions, values, agreements, and shared purpose. When we settle into transcendent Fulfillment, we are more Inspired (Virtue of Becoming), and we might very well see for the first-time other perspectives or concerns that we hadn't considered before, take that additional information into account, and have more profound transcendent Judgment (Polar Virtue) in terms of what is called for at that moment, all the while being more Forgiving and in that sense having No Judgement (other Polar Virtue).

From this transcendent perspective and as mentioned before regarding this and every Still Point, the reasoning of our subtle mind is supplemented and transformed by insights arising from Stillness. In a sense every Still Point is a portal to the Source, to the Absolute, to the Divine. The transcendent qualities that emerge from Source through all IPP Still Points can be summarized as Light (non-egoic discerning Wisdom), Love (without limit or qualification) and Life (High Vibrancy and Life Affirming) and Creativity, due to the inspiration of Light, Love and Live collectively transcending our existing constructs. In the process, as with every polarity, both polar qualities (lead/follow) which have fully flowed into one another, mutually embrace every situation with an effortless flow and facility informed by such Inspiration yielding more creative and flourishing outcomes.

Facilitation/Inquiry

In the more subtle variation of the concrete Purpose Polarity - facilitation/inquiry - there is by definition a more fluid, collaborative and ecosystemic approach to pursuing and exploring purpose and Possibility. This version of the Purpose Polarity arises most naturally at the top stage of the Subtle Tier of development ("Mature Integral") even as the basic Purpose Polarity initially arises at the top of the Concrete Tier. One of the markers of Mature Integral is to have an ability to work well with complex adaptive systems combined with the ecological awareness that tends to arise at the previous Early Integral stage, resulting in "ecosystemic" awareness and operational capacities in service of flourishing.

Resulting facilitative leadership tends to model "co-hosting" a group or ecosystem in a process whereby facilitation and inquiry are interpenetrating and fluid. The co-hosting quality is particularly relevant as we take account of the unique gifts, qualities, passions, purpose, and insights of the members of the group-ecosystem and integrate as best we can all the particular agencies-in-communion even as the individual members embrace the whole and contribute to communion-in-agency. Through this process we consciously, collaboratively, and creatively generate robust agreements in service of shared purposes and resulting outputs in service of interrelated individual and collective flourishing of the group and the ecosystems it serves.

In this context, one can summarize four important interrelated dimensions ("Four Primary Dimensions") to consider for optimizing the total value generated with regard to the net positive contributions to each of the multiple stakeholders in an ecosystem[21]: First, the culture and related underlying shared values and particularly the "agreements field" of a human ecosystem; Second, the structures and processes that support the ecosystem; Third, the moral, cognitive, and awareness qualities and capacities of members comprising the ecosystem specifically including that of the leadership collective; and Fourth, the be-

Integrative Purpose

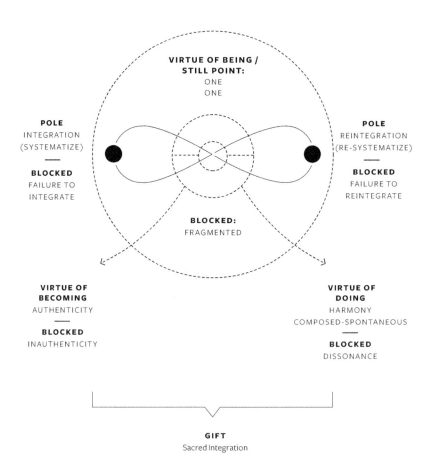

**VIRTUE OF BEING /
STILL POINT:**
ONE
ONE

POLE
INTEGRATION
(SYSTEMATIZE)

BLOCKED
FAILURE TO
INTEGRATE

POLE
REINTEGRATION
(RE-SYSTEMATIZE)

BLOCKED
FAILURE TO
REINTEGRATE

BLOCKED:
FRAGMENTED

**VIRTUE OF
BECOMING**
AUTHENTICITY

BLOCKED
INAUTHENTICITY

**VIRTUE OF
DOING**
HARMONY
COMPOSED-SPONTANEOUS

BLOCKED
DISSONANCE

GIFT
Sacred Integration

haviors and other outputs which arise. Prior to Mature Integral, most leaders (together with most evaluations and research orientations) tend to privilege one of those four dimensions, often ignoring the relevance or even existence of one or more of the others and are therefore at a significant disadvantage because unintended consequences arise when all four dimensions are not taken into consideration as "tetra arising" and mutually informing and influencing.

Integrative Purpose Polarity (integration/reintegration) also known as (systemization/re-systemization)

The primary IPP polarity that arises at the Mature Integral stage, which is fully complementary to the facilitation/inquiry version of the Purpose Polarity that also arises at Mature Integral, represents the quality of "purpose" related to the double "tier shift" up from intent (the Intent Polarity at the top of the Life Tier) and then purpose (the Purpose Polarity at the top of the Concrete Tier). It is designated as the "Integrative Purpose" polarity (integration/ reintegration).

There are integrative qualities at the top stage of every tier of development. They integrate all the qualities in that tier and provide a ground for the emergence of the next tier of development. However, this integrative quality is particularly significant at the top of the Subtle Tier - at Mature Integral. There is an integrative aspect associated with this stage of development and consciousness that for the first time tends to deeply honor and integrate the qualities of all prior stages of development within and among all of us more holistically in an ecosystemic context. This includes being able to more appreciatively recognize that all deeply held opinions - whether cultural or political - have elements of truth and expressions of authentic need or concern in them. Particularly with supportive training and ideally in the context of well-designed processes, such capacities increase the ability of people at this stage of maturity to weave together consensus-oriented solutions among those with highly diverse opinions and to achieve resolutions of even deep conflict, which is beyond the capacity of most people prior to this stage of development. For instance, Mature Integral capacities of facilitative leaders supported by IPP practices help to optimize flourishing outcomes of Connecting Conversations described previously.

In addition, a Flourishing Leader can adapt to leadership approaches and structures as needed in the circumstances. For instance, the hierarchical leadership structure of military organizations which reflects authority structures from the Concrete Tier of Development is necessary for many reasons, but such leadership and performance can be enriched and optimized by integrating many of the Mature Integral insights and approaches described here. In addition, just as leaders at Mature Integral can connect with people at every stage of development up to Mature Integral, they can also intuit how to work and negotiate optimally with other leaders and groups at various developmental stages in service of flourishing.

One challenge for many people with a Mature Integral developmental center of gravity is that having become, one might say, "masters" of the subtle thinking mind, they can become rather "fundamentalist" in the assumption that they feel that they have it "all figured out" through their mastery of the "subtle mind.". This can be reflected in having too many ready ecosystemic answers in every scenario. That is why the other pole to "integration" in this polarity is "reintegration," which creates the continual opening to new information and to greater complex adaptive, multi-ecosystemic restructuring and exploration[22]. This polar dynamic then includes being willing to take a perspective on our own assumptions and mental and operational models and systems, and systematically question, reframe and regenerate on an ongoing basis - even sometimes begin to live more comfortably in "Unknowing" which is a marker of moving into the Causal Tier of development.

In this spirit it is a co-responsibility of leadership for flourishing to be sure to uncover, honor and celebrate how each person and group defines their own flourishing. There is almost always a bias and often an unconscious one - cultural, developmental, scientific, etc. - that impacts my perspective regarding what I think flourishing is supposed to be for you. Variations of self-identified flourishing are extremely diverse, and as we are involved in leadership for flourishing, we should not only support others in clarifying and optimizing their self-defined flourishing but also learn from that and in the process potentially enrich our own understanding of flourishing by following in this regard as well as leading. This is a natural inclination at Mature Integral. *Nevertheless, a premise of IPP is that working toward an increasingly broader scope of love and caring awareness[23] and of ever deeper flourishing ecosystemic interconnectedness should be privileged as an underlying ethic of leadership for flourishing.*

As noted in Part 1, part of the IPP definition of flourishing includes flourishing regarding our ecosystemic interconnections, and the ecosystemic awareness related to the Mature Integral stage of development lends itself to further fleshing out the nature of flourishing in this regard. This ecosystemic approach to flourishing includes our physical, emotional, relational, moral, cognitive, and spiritual dimensions as involving "sub-ecosystems" of our overall individual human ecosystems and our capacity to resiliently generate flourishing of each such interconnected sub-ecosystems to contribute to the flourishing of our individual, collective and natural ecosystems. IPP polarities might be considered helpful simplified ecosystemic templates representing several of our human sub-ecosystems as we engage in facilitation/inquiry dynamics for our own internal flourishing as a primary element of IPP practice[24]. The flourishing of our personal human ecosystem is in turn profoundly interconnected with the flourishing of the ecosystems of human collectives of which each of us are a part, as well as being deeply interconnected with the flourishing of the broader ecosystems of the Life World and Material World in which we all co-exist.

This interpenetrating ecosystemic reality has been referred to as an "ontological connectedness."[25] Perhaps even beyond that, the Still Point of the Integrative Purpose Polarity is "One," that is, the transcendent quality that arises when the sense of integration of everything through the Integrative Purpose Polarity is complete, resulting in a sense of no separation: "All is One." From this place of deep Stillness and Oneness, we can begin to sense into cross paradigmatic possibilities beyond multi-systemic integrative cognitive processing which fully comes on line two stages later at the "Patterns Aware" stage in the Causal Tier of development.

There is a natural orientation of transcendent Authenticity (virtue of Becoming) that arises directly from that quality of Oneness rather than from one's Subtle Tier (most adults usual) self-sense. The Virtue of Doing that also naturally arises is transcendent Harmony. The transcendent Polar Virtues that arise from such Harmony are "Spontaneous" and "Composed." Harmony always arises Spontaneously out of the experience of Oneness, even as we Compose according to our specific purposes. These two transcendent qualities which both arise from the Harmony grounded in Oneness need each other in ongoing Creative Harmonic Emergence. Combining the IPP polarity and virtue practices related to the Mature Integral version of the Purpose Polarity (facilitation/exploration) grounded in Fulfillment and the Mature Integrative Purpose Polarity (integration/reintegration) grounded in Oneness is a potent foundation for deep and profound ecosystemic flourishing and transformation in the world.

There is another particularly relevant IPP polarity implicit in the foregoing that provides significant support for working in this ecosytemic context: ascending/descending (one of the four Foundational IPP polarities), which we call the Creation Polarity. The ascending dynamic relates to moving from the concreteness and current reality of things as they are, to a subtle flow of emotions and thoughts and entering into the causal Open Space of Possibility, Abundance, High Vibrancy, and potentially Creative New Vision. The other polar dynamic is "descending" in an ecologically embracing path from such Vision to the new subtle framing, to the creative concrete implementation. We then evaluate feedback and learn from that implementation in an ecosystemic context and continue in an ascending/descending polar cycle of implementing, learning more about flourishing from experience, re-visioning, and re-implementing - an endless regenerative dynamic in support of flourishing as our Wisdom deepens and contexts change. The Still Point of this polarity is the Wholeness of Creation.

A helpful metaphor developed by James Ritchie-Dunham affiliated with the Harvard Flourishing Network for framing this overall dynamic is that the concreteness of things is a noun, the subtle flow of the emotional and mental consciousness and energy is a verb, and innate Abundance opens up the potential for creativity and innovation. Then there is the embracing, ecological move of learning from the potential that was seen, manifested through verb into noun, providing feedback of what happened when we realize the potential which we envisioned. Through this cycle we can endlessly learn and evolve, changing the potential we see, the pathways of verbs to manifest the potential, and the noun-level concrete outputs those verbs generate regarding every context we address in our lives, organizations, communities[26].

Optimal leadership for flourishing is complex. It includes among other things working consciously and competently with the interrelated individual/collective, internal/external, local/global, Four Primary Dimensional, multi-ecosystemic, ascending/descending, aspects, and dynamics always at play. An inherent challenge is that people's scope of caring awareness as well as the degree of their awareness of and even capacity to grasp let alone work with such interrelated complexities is a function of their developmental stage of maturity. Deeply comprehending and being drawn to the importance of the interrelationships among these dimensions and dynamics arises initially at Mature Integral, and only a small minority of adults are at that stage of development - probably less than 5% but growing. Therefore, most families, organizations, businesses, communities, societies, etc. do not embrace assumptions values and agreements that reflect a concern or stewardship for let alone an ability to consciously and competently work with all these deeply interconnected ecosystemic elements of flourishing.

Attaining a critical mass of leaders in the world with at least Mature Integral capacities is desperately needed and ideally as many as possible with the centeredness and virtuous character attributes of Flourishing Leaders as the world is careening toward increasing conflict, institutional dysfunction, and ecological devastation. We need them to help bring us together in more Loving and flourishing families, organizations, communities, and nations in the context of more flourishing local/global ecologies.

The Rest of the Subtle Tier Polarities

When it comes to functioning with leadership for flourishing from the Mature Integral stage, which is the top stage of the Subtle Tier, it is also important to work well with the IPP polarities which represent primary polar dynamics that first arise at the prior three stages of the Subtle Tier. However, as is the case with any polarity that arises in the Subtle Tier, their polar dynamics move towards integration as we experience and work with them as we grow into the Mature Integral stage.

Expertise Polarity (assert knowledge/yield to knowledge)

The Expertise Polarity arises when we first grow into the first of four stages of the Subtle Tier of human development which we frame as being an "Early Modern" stage of development. A new subtle and more individualistic sense of identity arises at this stage, which includes an ability to think abstractly and to explore new ways of being in the world. One can understand and commit in a more comprehensive way to the universal principles found in national constitutions than one can at earlier stages. Yet the tendency at Early Modern is still to identify significantly with one's pre-existing groups and group-centric values which are deeply in place at the Mature Traditional Stage[27]. Those at

Expertise

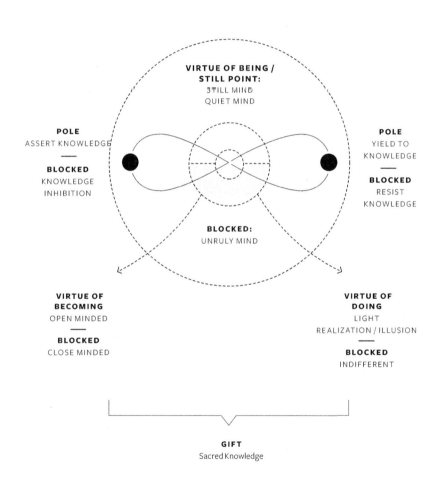

**VIRTUE OF BEING /
STILL POINT:**
STILL MIND
QUIET MIND

POLE
ASSERT KNOWLEDGE

BLOCKED
KNOWLEDGE
INHIBITION

POLE
YIELD TO
KNOWLEDGE

BLOCKED
RESIST
KNOWLEDGE

BLOCKED:
UNRULY MIND

**VIRTUE OF
BECOMING**
OPEN MINDED
—
BLOCKED
CLOSE MINDED

**VIRTUE OF
DOING**
LIGHT
REALIZATION / ILLUSION
—
BLOCKED
INDIFFERENT

GIFT
Sacred Knowledge

Early Modern then, are particularly adept at using their complex thinking abilities and sometimes cherry picking their facts to defend their group-centric world views, taking an ideological position, and defending it. They tend to see others who believe differently than they do as somehow defective, in part because they have a challenging time grasping points of view other than their own. In times of low trust and polarization in society there is a significant risk that a substantial portion of people at Early Modern will "pull in" even more tightly to the perceived safety of their group centric (Mature Traditional) commitments and beliefs inconsistent with universal principles, science, and mature rationality. We are seeing increasing amounts of this phenomenon in the early 21st century which is experiencing so much uncertainty and institutional dysfunction.

There is a tendency at the Early Modern stage of development to lean towards being a perfectionist and to master a skill or a discipline; yet people at early modern have difficulty prioritizing goals and time. There are many highly intelligent and skilled individuals at this stage of development who become leaders in professional and academic disciplines, where unambiguous expertise is particularly important, although many people at significantly higher stages of development may chose similar careers.

When the Expertise Polarity (assert knowledge/yield to knowledge) first arises then, a person at this early modern stage of development tends to hold subtle forms of knowledge such as abstract ideas and concepts rigidly - often dogmatically - in a tight conceptual framework and resists yielding to new knowledge other than from experts or authority figures whom they recognize. From the second stage of development in the Subtle Tier, "Mature Modern" one tends to look at various alternatives more freely and choose one based on "either/or" thinking. The conclusion tends to be that there is one best answer. Then at the third or "Early Integral" stage of development in the Subtle Tier, people begin to see "both/and" possibilities, realizing that everyone has perspectives that are valuable even if such perspectives may seem inconsistent. So, in the context of this polarity someone at Early Integral can hold and value asserting knowledge and receiving knowledge fluidly and contemporaneously but often without a significant capacity for synthesizing multiple seeming inconsistencies. At the Mature Integral stage of development, greater integrative capacities come online, and there is tendency to integrate the process of receiving and asserting knowledge, often yielding new emergent possibilities, and yet also often valuing paradox.

As we move beyond Mature Integral into the next four stage tier of development - the Causal Tier - we become more aware in the moment that as we receive new information, we are framing it and testing it in the context of our existing knowledge constructs. As we come to notice the limitations of the constructions of our own understanding, we are more open to new possibilities. The approach in IPP practice for working with those in the Subtle Tier of development (which in the developed world includes the vast majority of adults) is initially to support them in moving toward the Mature Integral processing of the subtle thinking mind and related awareness of local/global eco-systemic interconnectedness, as supplemented by drawing on deeper transcendent and intuitive qualities - which as mentioned previously we summarize as Light, Love, Life and Creativity - which flow through IPP Still Points. Support is then provided for growing into the Causal Tier of development.

The Still Point Virtue of Being of asserting knowledge/receiving knowledge - the experience of the transcendent "Still Mind" - is a meditative accomplishment but does not mean that you stop using the subtle thinking mind. As we settle into that Still Point quality, we become more Open Minded (Virtue of Becoming) to supplementing and informing subtle thinking processes with the intuitive Light (Virtue of Doing) that flows from Source through the portal of the Still Mind and which generates as well qualities of transcendent Love, Life and Creativity. The transcendent polarities that emerge out of Light - Realization and Illusion - help us appreciate that a deeper, richer "Realization" of reality and possibility arises out of the Light, and at the same time we are aware that any framing of that reality is ultimately partial - an "Illusion." Nevertheless, progress is made by continually reassessing and connecting to a deeper reality by being Open to Light and Possibility through deep inner Stillness and Quietness in the context of asserting and receiving knowledge.

The good news is that by IPP practice relating to knowledge always moving to the transcendent qualities of Stillness, Openness, Light, Realization and Illusion, if the proper processes and system design are put in place, supported by adequately trained and mature leadership, an open, creative and generative learning community can be established without participants themselves needing to master Mature Integral cognitive processes. Ironically, these "sophisticated" structures and processes enable and support the simplicity and naturalness of the way children play and learn together.

The IPP polar and virtue qualities of this polarity are supportive of any learning and knowledge sharing environment, but they can be exemplified particularly well in formal educational environments. Practicing these virtues supports a learning community environment, where there is no ego need to be "right." There is a natural playfulness that arises, and one explores the interface and inter-weaving of what we know, what we do not know, what we are learning, and emergent possibilities. When such a learning community environment is held in Trust and Love, the inclusive process of collective inquiry becomes an exercise in interrelated individual, collective and ecosystemic flourishing.

Regarding a formal teaching environment, the emphasis is initially tending to an ascending hierarchy of needs. First, the concrete essentials of *Life*, such as food, shelter, and safety are foundational for learning. "Trust" is a pre-condition for a healthy and productive learning community and in a deeper sense invites *Love*. Love is a precondition for optimal learning. Even if Love is often missing in a formal sense in educational settings, caring and loving teachers and administrators who often get little recognition for those qualities of character and heart are more numerous in our schools than we ever give them credit for. Love not only opens up all of us for greater learning and more *Light*; this evolutionary trajectory draws us into the open space of creativity and other full spectrum growth, integration, and transformation, that is, into the fullness of our Beings - into the fullness of flourishing[28].

One of the leading scholars, researchers and practitioners of flourishing, Matthew T. Lee, PhD has utilized an open space environment in higher education that might more typically be seen in a kindergarten setting where there is "open space for friendship, care, joy, creativity, agency, deep engagement and the experience of flourishing in multiple domains."[29] This open space model emphasizes the integration of cognitive, affective, and experiential forms of learning in a context of freedom and creativity. Dr. Lee emphasizes that this is a "love-based technology of change" based on the observation that all of us flourish in non-instrumental spaces in which we feel safe and cared for and also have agency to explore without unnecessary limits. Note the alignment of the principles in this and the previous paragraph with principles of healthy attachment and the Foundational Patterns of Leadership for Flourishing imbedded in the Relations Polarity. As Dr. Lee puts it, he is describing how to create the conditions for collective emergent learning and inquiry and "loving people into being" and practicing "to enact a new world."

Such enactment is the polar dynamic counterpoint to the creative evolutionary impulse. It constitutes ecologically "involving" or descending from *Light* and possibility to *Love* and *Life* affirming *Creative* engagement holistically creating a new world grounded in *Freedom, Love* and *Flourishing*. One important framing element embedded in the IPP ecosystem in this regard is a conscious involutionary trajectory as follows:

- "Light" is the Virtue of Doing of the Expertise Polarity, the most involutionary polarity of the Subtle Tier;
- "Love" is the Virtue of Doing of the most involutionary polarity of the Concrete Tier;

- "Life" is the Virtue of Doing of the most involutionary polarity of the Life Tier;
- Holistic and Creative "Unique Compassionate Embrace" of Light, Love, and Life together with the transcendent polar output of Freedom and Love is the Virtue of Doing of the most involutionary and ecologically embracing polarity of the entire IPP ecosystem[30].

The evolutionary trajectory embraces the same themes in ascending order. The spirit of the ascending/descending polar dynamics of what we call the Fullness of Creation polarity aligns deeply with Dr. Lee's vision of "enacting a new world."

Stabilizing in the Still Point of Quite Mind and being transcendently Open Minded (Virtue of Becoming) and Sourcing Light (Virtue of Doing) beyond the more normal subtle mind in the context of experiencing the integration of the poles of subtle IPP polarities supports one in transitioning into the Causal Tier of Development. When one is ready, practicing the initial "Construct Aware" Causal Tier polarity (language meaning/empty language) supports one in working with a new appreciation that language and all our subtle knowledge frameworks and boundaries are constructs. There are deeper and more intuitive patterns that underlie Subtle Tier knowledge that include but subtly transform and interconnect subtle knowledge constructs in ways that are previously unimaginable through the "subtle mind." Fully grasping and having facility in working with such patterns arises at the next stage of the Causal Tier through the Kosmic Patterning polarity briefly described later in this book - even as Causal Consciousness itself helps us rest in the Beauty of Unknowing.

Achievement (subjectification/objectification)

The next emergent stage of development beyond Early Modern, which

Achievement

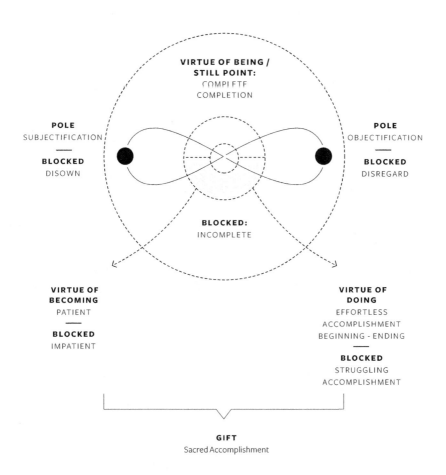

**VIRTUE OF BEING /
STILL POINT:**
COMPLETE
COMPLETION

POLE
SUBJECTIFICATION

BLOCKED
DISOWN

POLE
OBJECTIFICATION

BLOCKED
DISREGARD

BLOCKED:
INCOMPLETE

**VIRTUE OF
BECOMING**
PATIENT
—
BLOCKED
IMPATIENT

**VIRTUE OF
DOING**
EFFORTLESS
ACCOMPLISHMENT
BEGINNING - ENDING
—
BLOCKED
STRUGGLING
ACCOMPLISHMENT

GIFT
Sacred Accomplishment

we call "Mature Modern," and when the Achievement Polarity becomes particularly relevant, is a more fully developed and integrated manifestation of the Early Modern stage of development. The cognitive capacities related to the Mature Modern stage gave birth to the Enlightenment. People at this stage of development tend to be goal oriented with a much greater capacity and inclination to set and follow through on priorities in an orderly manner than those at Early Modern, which is of course an extremely helpful leadership capacity. There is a new ability to see common qualities in all people which for instance often generates a commitment to human rights. Even as they often support such universal principles, those at Mature Modern tend to prioritize those commitments only within their own nation state, typically the largest collective with which they deeply identify. Developing Mature Modern cognitive and moral capacities has for the most part been the goal of most educational systems in the West for the past few centuries.

Mature Modern leaders have been responsible for enormous global advances in the spread of learning, civilization, and economic prosperity over the past two hundred years. They have also led us to the cusp of global environmental devastation because at this stage of development there is typically not a grasp of the nature of local/global ecosystems and how much they are deeply interconnected and how humans are imbedded within them. In addition, Mature Modern leaders and institutions have been increasingly failing to deal adequately with the complexity of twenty first century realities. As previously noted, the large majority of adults in the developed world are somewhere in the range of Early Modern to Mature Modern stages of development.

The subjectification/objectification polarity reflects a primary Mature Modern polar tension resulting from the concreteness and broad polar separation of the concepts of "subject" and "object" at this stage of development. That distinct separation optimizes the prominence of the subtle identity at this stage in the Subtle Tier of development and leverages the observational and analytical powers of the formal operational cognitive capacities associated with the Mature Modern stage. By shifting the concreteness of "subject" and "object" to the more fluid qualities of "subjectification" and "objectification" in IPP practice, the multiple aspects of our identities become more evident, and we can see more clearly how understanding multiple aspects in others helps us clarify our own qualities of personhood, which is often called "intersubjective awareness.". This phenomenon begins to appear naturally at the next stage of development: Early Integral.

As we facilitate the integration of subjectification and objectification, which begins to happen naturally at Mature Integral, those facilitated begin to see and feel the ecosystemic local/global webs of connections among all sentient beings and nature. We also begin to see that our subjective framing in a sense creates the objects that are being objectified through the subjectification-objectification polar dynamic. There is a seed of the subject in the object and of the object in the subject. It should be noted though, that there is such deep attachment for most of us to the subtle subject - the subtle sense of self - that this is a particularly difficult polarity to move fully into integration and beyond. Through IPP practice when we drop into the Still Point Virtue of Being, Transcendent Completion, where subjectification and objectification are no longer two, an experience of sharing "interbeing"[31] - related to a sense of underlying oneness - with other people often occurs, sometimes with regard to all other sentient beings, and even with all manifestation.

When the Still Point of this polarity, Completion, is stabilized, the drive to achieve associated with the Mature Modern stage of development transforms. From the place of the Abundance of Completion we no longer feel driven to achieve goals from a position of chronic deficit. However as with every IPP Virtue of Being, the paradox exists that through the experience of bringing the poles into a unified Stillness, the capacity is amplified to engage in the moment with deeper Intuition and greater flow and efficacy in the relevant bandwidth of consciousness, energy and function, thereby in this instance with the Achievement Polarity of increasing our capacity to achieve desired ends.

This involves transcendent "Effortless Accomplishment" (the relevant Virtue of Doing) accompanied by transcendent Patience (the relevant Virtue of Becoming). "Effortless Accomplishment" is framed as such because there is no ego striving involved, where results emerge from holding intention and purpose, being in flow and being supported by other virtuous qualities of character. The related Virtue of Becoming, Patience, is also a particularly helpful transcendent quality of character because when we experience it and practice it, we for instance find ourselves moving beyond egoic competitiveness, the need for social or hierarchical approval, and being concerned about self-imposed time frames that don't match the actual requirements of the realities of the situation being addressed.

As mentioned previously we often refer to such IPP Virtues of Doing and Becoming collectively as transcendent "Character Virtues" because they are non-egoic qualities of character arising from the deep Stillness of Being (Virtue of Being). Although generally described as a polarity practice which draws us toward greater flow, integration and over time growth, IPP is also often characterized as a virtue practice, which emphasizes transcendent qualities of virtuous character arising out of Virtues of Being in the context of each stage of our human development. It is both.

When people are facilitated into these Character Virtues in IPP practice they typically share their own unique insights and expressions of those Virtues, but based on working with the many hundreds of people the author has facilitated over more than the past twenty years, those being facilitated almost always describe the same universal transcendent essence related to each respective Character Virtue, even without having previously been provided a description of those qualities. They are simply already there waiting to be awakened. During facilitations of a particular Character Virtue, frequently other Character Virtues "speak up" and bring forward complementary qualities and perspectives. Particularly the Character Virtues arising out of the same Virtue of Being ("Related Character Virtues") tend to want to "speak up" in tandem - in this instance, Patience and Effortless Accomplishment. We find that other Character Virtue combinations arise frequently. For instance, Hope and Patience are particularly supportive of one another. The Related Character Virtues that seem to be most pervasively present and influential no matter what other Character Virtues are being addressed are the Character Virtues of the Relations Polarity: Love and Hope[32]. As previously noted, Love is the lubricant which interconnects and informs all other Character Virtues in their shared contribution to flourishing, and Hope is an attitude which among other things enables us to hold well whatever we lovingly encounter in life.

We are always looking for approaches to character and virtues which reflect similar transcendent sensibilities, and relationships such as those described above, to further learn and be enriched and inspired by the power and beauty of their expression. One excellent example comes from Edward Brooks DPhil, executive director of the Oxford Character Project, and one of the leading scholars on character and virtues and particularly the virtue of Hope. Brooks gives elegant voice to such interconnections of Patience, Hope and Love in his description of what he calls "good hope":

> Hope is receptive, it involves a certain way of seeing the world, its provisionality, its pain, and its promise. And it is lived in a mode of patient waiting, towards a future that cannot be manufactured. And yet we are not simply to wait around. If virtue is formed in practice, we can learn the 'art', or skill, of good hope by practices of receptivity: waiting without immediately seeking diversion; enduring difficulty whilst resisting the resolution offered by presumption or despair; listening without jumping to conclusions; looking with the awareness that there is always more than meets the eye; appreciating others without succumbing to the pressure to compete; being where we are and being thankful for it; committing to live beyond ourselves because love has a future[33].

In this context Dr. Brooks references Emily Dickenson's metaphor that "hope is the thing with feathers that perches the soul – And sings the tune without words – And never stops at all." He goes on to say that: "like a bird, hope may be small, but it is also hardy. The lightness of its presence belies a strength that keeps it singing through life's most powerful storms. That challenge when it comes to growing in hope is to learn to listen: to tune in – And then to join in – the song."

Dr. Brooks holds the paradoxical polar insight that that passive patience of good hope also engenders active perseverance beyond normal human inclination as it "never stops at all" and "engages in the song." We find that in IPP practice a common expression of transcendent Patience invites the co-participation of transcendent Perseverance.

As noted previously, the IPP Virtue of Being, out of which both Hope and Love arise is transcendent Trust. Such Hope is beyond hoping for things (a vice of attachment in the Buddhist tradition) or most other definitions of hope. It is rather through Grace, one might say in the Christian tradition, or some deep non-egoic quality of Spirit or Being arising out of Trust which gives this "good hope" its distinct and transcendent character and its deeply symbiotic association with transcendent Love and its many related qualities such as transcendent Loving Kindness, Empathy, Compassion, and Joy.

The Oxford Character Project[34] takes the position that character is the core of responsible leadership committed to human flourishing which among other research-based qualities of character highlights the importance of Hope, Gratitude, Empathy, Love and Compassion - all deeply imbedded in IPP practice. A key in understanding the connection of character and leadership in support of flourishing is to appreciate that developing "good character" is foundational to human flourishing itself. There is increasingly research which concludes that good character - specifically including love and caring - contributes profoundly to human flourishing, as summarized for instance in a December 2022 research update by Tyler J. Vander Weele, Director of the Harvard University Human Flourishing Program at the Harvard's Institute for Quantitative Social Science[35]. He says thatleaders should model and inspire flourishing for others through their own good character as well as develop character strengths and related skills that specifically support the flourishing of others such as the virtues and skills related to aligning with and creating clarity around elevated shared purpose as is explored in the last previous section of this Part 2. IPP is a character and virtue practice particularly supportive of such endeavors.

There are important research- based approaches to highly effective leadership for flourishing grounded in good character. One particularly impressive example which reflects an elegant simplicity on the other side of a great deal of research-based complexity is the book, *Leader; Know Love and Inspire your People*[36]. For instance, the book emphasizes the importance of leaders getting to know those they lead through Empathetic listening and grounding their leadership in Love. It stresses the importance of connecting the values of those we lead to the purpose of the organization and in turn to an even broader, nobler cause. The book emphasizes many other key elements of character, particularly of learning to put in hard work and developing grit and perseverance aligned with the passion and values and shared purpose of those in the organizations that we lead. It also emphasizes the importance of being deeply Hopeful and Patient in the context of Perseverance. Among other things, this book explicates with wonderful examples almost all of the Foundational Patterns of Leadership for Flourishing.

The authors, Katy Granville-Chapman, and Emmie Bidston, exemplify their book's message. They are both research fellows at the Oxford Character Project, co-chair the Harvard/Oxford Leadership for Flourishing Community of Practice affiliated with Harvard University's Human Flourishing Program at Harvard's Institute for Quantitative Social Science and are Senior Fellows of The Human Flourishing Program's Flourishing Network. Katy Granville-Chapman, who received a Doctorate from Oxford University, among other things is a Doctoral Teaching Fellow at Oxford University's Department of Education,; a Research Associate at the Oxford University Wellbeing Research Centre,; and a co-founder of and deeply engaged in Global Social Leaders, (a movement of young people in 105 countries who design and lead social action projects that make a meaningful change in their communities). Emmie Bidston studied Economics at the University of Cambridge and among other things is currently head of Economics at Wellington College, Director of the Wellington Leadership and Coaching Institute, and is deeply engaged in a charity that helps develop young leaders in Africa. She also runs conferences, coaching, and leadership training for adults and young people. In short, such extensive involvements and accomplishments of these two women do not arise out of egoic efforting, but rather from sterling qualities of character and virtuous commitments, particularly including leadership through love and the interconnected flourishing of us all. That is simply who they are[37].

Some wonderful leadership as well as research and scholarship around character-based leadership in education is also originating from the Virtue and Values Education Center ("VVEC") of the Universidad Francisco de Vitoria in Madrid Spain under the leadership of Veronica Fernández Espinosa. Dr. Fernández also serves as a consultant for the Values Based Leadership Project of the Oxford Character Project. She co-authored an article entitled "The Effects of Teacher Leadership on Students' Purposeful Learning,"[38] regarding research sponsored by VVEC, which highlights five leadership traits of teachers that their research suggests are particularly impactful in supporting student and as well as teacher flourishing: empathetic leadership, comforting leadership, motivational leadership, wise leadership, and exemplar leadership. The first two modalities of leadership address the importance of the teacher or leader being in Communion with students grounded in Appropriate, Trusting, and Caring relationships. The second two modalities relate to the importance of purposeful learning aligned with shared virtues and values. The last modality of leadership -exemplar leadership - stresses how important it is for teachers to inspire students by modeling whom they would encourage their students to become. These principles are deeply resonant with the research and work relating to virtuous leadership and education of Brooks and Granville-Chapman/ Bidston referenced in this section, as well with as the patterns of IPP.

Context Aware (contextualization/deconstruction)

The Early Integral stage of development, when the Context Aware Polarity first arises became culturally significant in the second half of the 20th century, when for the first time a critical mass of adults in the developed world grew into a center of gravity at this stage and began to materially transform national and global cultures. From this developmental "altitude" there is a natural ability to not just take a deeper perspective on many of the assumptions of modernism (and thereby to appreciate how everyone's views are significantly socially constructed). People at this stage of development also perceive that our perspectives are conditioned by endless contexts. This often leads to an emphasis on deconstructing the institutions, hierarchies, values and world view of group-centric and modern people and cultures, but usually without the capacity to replace them with a more adequate framework.

There is also a new also a new capacity to see internal contexts and sensitivities at this stage. When combined with the phenomenon that consistent with each early stage of development is more passive and receptive than those at mature stages, such those at Mature Integral, those at Early Integral have a heightened sensitivity to being offended when those around them are not being sensitive to all their and others' multiple dimensions of sensitivity. As such those at Early Integral become particularly concerned about those who are marginalized, and whose sensitivities have previously been ignored or suppressed. When these concerns are formalized there arises an ethos of what is often referred to as "political correctness." The extensive lists in many higher education settings in the United States of banned offensive language and "micro-agressions" is an expression of such political correctness. In such settings, many students but also sometimes faculty and staff - par-

Context Aware

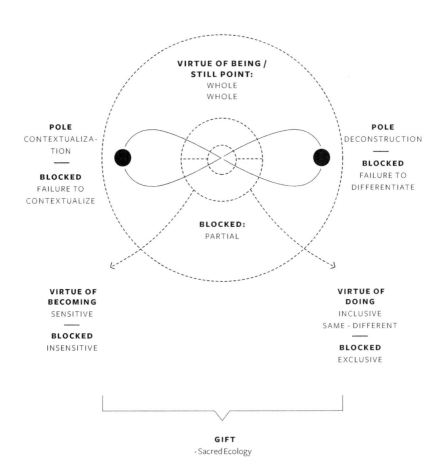

**VIRTUE OF BEING /
STILL POINT:**
WHOLE
WHOLE

POLE
CONTEXTUALIZA-
TION
—
BLOCKED
FAILURE TO
CONTEXTUALIZE

POLE
DECONSTRUCTION
—
BLOCKED
FAILURE TO
DIFFERENTIATE

BLOCKED:
PARTIAL

**VIRTUE OF
BECOMING**
SENSITIVE
—
BLOCKED
INSENSITIVE

**VIRTUE OF
DOING**
INCLUSIVE
SAME - DIFFERENT
—
BLOCKED
EXCLUSIVE

GIFT
‹ Sacred Ecology

ticularly those who are not yet at an Early Integral stage - accept these standards as dogma and enact extreme intolerance toward (insensitivity to) and even rejection of those who are not adequately politically correct. This is a sensitivity performative contradiction to which many early integralists are blind.

Such Early Integral deconstruction and political correctness can be mystifying and offensive to those who are Modern and Traditional, and as noted the early integralists tend not to be very tolerant of those with Traditional and Modern world views and "insensitivities." This can lead to mutual misunderstanding, and resentment, and to an implosion to group-centric, resentful, dogmatic attitudes and actions - of people and groups on both on the right and the left culturally and politically, which has become increasingly prevalent in the 21st century.

The Mature Integral response to Modern and Traditional insensitivities and Early Integral hypersensitivities tends to be more one of curiosity and empathy and attempting to connect with, love, and embrace people from all personal and cultural backgrounds and developmental altitudes. We desperately need societal leadership with such maturity who can model these qualities and share more effectively that a flourishing society necessarily requires not only a recognition of universal rights and responsibilities but a loving and compassionate embrace of all.

Since those with an Early Integral developmental center of gravity tend to reject hierarchies - typically assuming that all hierarchies are inappropriately based primarily on power - they often tend to reject the idea that there are healthy and helpful developmental hierarchies, particularly that they themselves represent a less mature version (Early Integral) of a next stage of development (Mature Integral). They often hold the perspective that their views are superior to all others (including those of Mature Integral) – an unacknowledged hierarchical assumption asserted inconsistently with a stated anti-hierarchical worldview. Nevertheless, many people at Early Integral are inclusive and collaborative and appreciative of all people, particularly in dialogical environments, which qualities and capacities come more fully into fruition at Mature Integral.

It is especially helpful if those at Early Integral begin to appreciate that there is another half step of maturity that they can grow into and be guided to some extent by the more mature capacities and perspectives of Mature Integral. Arising at this "both/and" third stage of the Subtle Tier of development (the third stage of all three tiers in the Human World manifest a both/and sensibility), it is an important practice with the contextualization/deconstruction polarity to experience the integration of these two qualities that occurs naturally at Mature Integral. This integration involves an endless dynamic of deconstructing the ultimately limited constructed frameworks of the mind and simultaneously re-constructing them in more inclusive ecosystemic contexts – and through the portal of the Still Point informed by deeper intuitions and patterns.

Since at Early Integral we open up more fully to the multiple contexts and aspects within ourselves, the "voice dialogue" technique often used in IPP of speaking to various temporal and transcendent aspects within each of us and among all of us tends to become more impactful than for those at earlier stages of development[39]. As previously noted by doing inner work through IPP or through other therapeutic means, we inevitably uncover elements within us that are repressed, perhaps manifesting pathologically, which can be worked on by what is often called "shadow work." Through voice dialogue or otherwise, IPP is a practice that helps every aspect within us become more transparent, functional, and interconnected and source the inner wisdom that resides in that bandwidth of ourselves.

As noted previously IPP polarities function as sub-ecosystems within our personal ecosystems where we can say that inner ecosystemic shadow work is important. This orientation also helps us be more conscious as well of the importance of shadow work in our ecosystemic work in the world. For instance, there are frequently "shadow" sub-ecosystems of abuse embedded within many institutional ecosystems that generate institutional silence and protect perpetrators of even serious abuse, such as sexual abuse, including those institutions overtly committed by their own policies to protect the vulnerable[40]. A crucial element of leadership for flourishing should be to do the "institutional shadow work" of helping to identify institutional abuse, to ensure transparency and accountability in the event of such abuse, and to work to eliminate the organizational sub-ecosystems that enable abuse. In the long run the goal is to support individual and group flourishing in the context of healing, restoration, and regeneration, but in the short term, there may need to be some "tough love" and even legal recourse to get difficult situations resolved and insidious shadow ecosystems eliminated.

The Virtue of Being of the Early Integral polarity, "Wholeness," brings to Stillness the overall dynamic of this contextualization/deconstruction polarity which is always reaching toward Wholeness without quite getting there and opens us up to profound and Sacred Wholeness in every moment. Identifying deeply with such Wholeness enables us to heal from the fragmentation and woundedness that we all experience in life much more effectively and holistically than if we begin solely from a place of deficit.

We facilitate another type of conversation grounded in a facilitated experience of Wholeness which can build on the Healing nature of a Connecting Conversation experience. We call it a "Healing Conversation." When people in a group are facilitated into an experience of Wholeness, it is for most people a remarkable moment, because most of us are so accustomed particularly in the context of deep division and even hostility to coming from deficit, fragmentation, and even woundedness. The Healing Conversations experience is comprised essentially of people coming together in a spirit of Healing to share their experience of being personally challenged or wounded from the difficulties of dealing with a challenging issue or experience. In a container of Trust, Love, and Wholeness, we listen deeply and empathetically to one another and hold one another in a spirit of Compassion and Healing - not as advocates of a position on an issue but as fellow human beings in Sacred Communion, loving one another into Healing and Wholeness even as Sacred Wholeness holds us all.

The Still point of "Wholeness" of the Early Integral polarity has an important polar and harmonic relationship to the Still Point of "Oneness" of the Mature Integral polarity. These two Still Point qualities - Oneness and Wholeness - are two transcendent framing qualities that add an important transcendent dimension to the IPP Harmonic described in Part 1[41]. When we come from Oneness there is a natural Harmonic Beauty that emerges. When we come from Wholeness, we experience Healing and the Sacred. These two transcendent qualities (or "Transcendent Notes") - Oneness and Wholeness - frame three core themes ("Core Temporal Notes"): the "stillness" or "causal,", the "flowing" or "subtle,", and the "concrete," which represent collectively in various manifestations the full spectrum of consciousness, energy and function of the pervasive temporal and fleeting qualities of our lives. This "chord" of the IPP Harmonic then, is comprised of three Core Temporal Notes framed by two Transcendent Notes: "One, still, flow, concrete, Whole."

When the two Transcendent Notes fully flow into one another, they can be summarized as the experience of "Sacred Beauty." Without the fleeting temporal dimensions of our experience being held in Sacred Beauty, we are often deeply burdened sometimes even overwhelmed by the vicissitudes of life. However, if these temporal qualities are experienced in the context of Sacred Beauty, we can be uplifted from moment to moment. Through this Harmonic we play endless variations of the jazz composition of our lives as an experience of Sacred Beauty. In this context, IPP can be summarized as a practice of learning to live, love, and lead in Sacred Beauty.

This framing of the fleeting nature of our lives in the context of experiencing Harmony arising out of Oneness and healing out of Wholeness is resonant with a Japanese aesthetic: in every moment appreciate a profound Harmony arising out of Oneness and heal from holding the Wholeness of experience. This aesthetic is also deeply connected to the natural world, reflective of the deep alignment with Sacred Nature found in of the Japanese Shinto spiritual tradition.

A profound integrative therapy grounded in this Japanese aesthetic has been co-developed by Japanese naturopathic physician Mami Ishii ND, affiliated with the Harvard Flourishing Network, and her colleague Ted Lo MD, a Chinese psychiatrist. This "delicious moment" therapy ("DLM") emphasizes a pervasive Japanese metaphor of "Savoring" each Sacred Moment. DLM utilizes this tradition of healing through Sacred Beauty in the context of western allopathic and naturopathic medicine and psychotherapy, where one learns to savor one's authentic beauty to heal and flourish. The DLM therapeutic approach works with the full spectrum of our beings - body, emotions, mind, soul, and spirit - and "opens clients to experience unconditional love into the transcending opportunity of hope, meaning and purpose"[42].

This tradition of living in Sacred Beauty is also reminiscent of the Native American Navajo Sacred tradition of deeply connecting to the natural world and similarly valuing the centrality of Beauty in every moment. For instance, following is one of many variations of a prayer in a Navajo blessing ceremony:

With Beauty before me I walk.
With Beauty behind me I walk.
With Beauty above me I walk.
With Beauty around me I walk.
In Beauty I walk.

Ramona Sierra, a Navajo traditional healer, and licensed therapist, brings this Sacred Beauty into her therapeutic healing practice, working to bring Beauty and Wholeness into the lives particularly of those who have experienced severe trauma[43]. Her therapeutic work of bringing abused animals (especially horses) and traumatized people together in their shared vulnerability to heal one another through a shared instinct for loving one another into Healing and Wholeness is a deep work of Sacred Beauty.

The Navajo educator, Clayton Long, clarifies that the Navajo "Beauty Way" or "Blessing Way" (Hozho) represents the interconnection of all life and being, which calls all of us to love, peace, understanding and joy. He notes that we (all people, all life, the earth) must learn to heal together so that we do not die together. His parents told him that in their lifetime the world was still not yet ready to listen to this message. He suggests and hopes in this moment where we live on the edge of global environmental disaster that the world is finally ready for this wisdom, and he has committed his life to sharing this message[44].

In a higher "register" of the IPP Harmonic Chord there is a transcendent expression of the three Core Temporal Notes comprised of the Transcendent qualities of Light (from still or causal), Love (from flowing or subtle), and Life (from concrete) (collectively, Transcendent Core Notes) creating a fully transcendent expression of the IPP Harmonic Chord: "One, Light, Love, Life, Whole". Another expression of this is that when the framing transcendent Notes of Oneness and Wholeness fully flow into one another and become "Not-Two," "Sacred Beauty" is inspired and directed in the moment through the flow of the three Transcendent Core Notes of transcendent Wisdom (Light); unqualified and unlimited loving kindness, empathy and, compassion (Love); in modalities that support and respect the Lives of each of us interconnected with Lives of all of us including the natural world (Life) expressed in utterly unique and creative ways depending on our individual and collective circumstances and Gifts (Creativity). These are the transcendent qualities that flow through every IPP polarity Still Point and which deeply inform us from moment to moment as we live in Sacred Beauty.

The epicenter of this five note transcendent Harmonic Chord - One, Light, Love, Life, Whole – is Love. As stressed throughout this book, Love is the very essence of flourishing. We come to understand that Sacred Beauty is by definition grounded in Love. Sacred Beauty is a capstone of the IPP framing for life and leadership in support of flourishing. In the spirit of "as with the inner, the outer", we recognize that in our families, organizations, communities and ecosystemic interconnectedness (local all the way to global) there is pervasive fragmentation and woundedness, and that by coming from a place of Wholeness which embraces all with Love, shared Sacred Healing can take place. Also, when we come from Oneness, what emerges through Light, Love and Life to address our shared challenges in the world is Harmonious and Beautiful. Let us learn to Savor each moment that we may have an opportunity to Love one another into Healing and Wholeness as an expression of Sacred Beauty. A conversation grounded in this Sacred aesthetic - a Conversation of Sacred Beauty - can build on the healing nature of the Healing Conversations experience and generate inspired solutions to our most pressing problems.

The Causal Tier of Human Development

There are likely less than one percent of adults who have stabilized in any of the four stages of the Causal Tier of human development, and each successive stage of development within the Causal Tier is increasingly rare. Nevertheless, those who have stabilized at the second or "Kosmic Patterning Aware" stage in the Causal Tier (Kosmic Patterning polarity: Witnessing/ Kosmic Patterns) tend to have significant additional capacities of transformational leadership beyond what is possible in the Subtle Tier of development culminating with Mature Integral. A person with a Kosmic Patterning Aware developmental center of gravity can sense deep patterns, interconnections, and possibilities across diverse disciplines in philosophy, the arts and the sciences that previously seemed unrelated and tends to design, plan, and strategize for global impact over multiple generations.

Although rare, there are clearly some people coming from at least a Kosmic Patterning Aware developmental center of gravity who are already implementing profound original approaches to addressing local/global issues with exceptional qualities of freshness, Abundance, and Possibility. Perhaps the most prominent early example as described in Part 1 is Ken Wilber's overlaying the internal/external polarity at a 90 degree angle over the individual/collective polarity to reveal for the first time that virtually every science, philosophy, and point of view, arises primarily out of one of the resulting four quadrants (referred to previously as the Four Primary Dimensions), and then combining that insight with the integration of stages of development and other factors in his integral philosophy. It can be argued that this seemingly very simple "integral" framework created a meta-perspective beyond all the prior categorizing perspectives. Wilber's extensive writings have also inspired a great deal of "integrally informed" research and applications in multiple disciplines over the past few decades.

Kosmic Patterning Aware theorists and activists move beyond the body/mind integration seen at Mature Integral and include the powerful sourcing of deeper causal awareness, inspiration, and creativity – one might say the integration of body/mind/spirit. One can see these sensibilities in the work of Otto Scharmer affiliated with MIT and leader of the Presencing Institute previously mentioned. In his landmark book *Theory U: Leading From The Future As It Emerges*[45] he shares an approach that systematizes how groups can optimize planning and decision making by experiencing the dramatic re-framing that can result from sourcing inspiration beyond the thinking mind. In terms of leadership, they talk about "leading from the future": Building upon decades of action research at MIT, the process shows how "individuals, teams, organizations, and large systems can build the essential leadership capacities needed to address the root causes of today's social, environmental, and spiritual challenges." As they express it, they show how to update the "operating code" in our societal systems through a shift in consciousness from ego-system to "eco-system awareness."

Those at the particularly mature manifestations of the Kosmic Patterning Aware stage and beyond sometimes develop approaches which grasp the simplicity beyond Mature Integral multi-systemic complexity, reach deeply and transformationally into our more foundational polarities to turn things on their head and identify seemingly simple and radically effective approaches to our complex challenges. James Ritchie-Dunham provides an example of this. With Bettye Pruitt he authored *Econsynomics: – The Science of Abundance*[46], which posits a theory of economics based on Abundance rather than scarcity, (the foundation of all previous prominent economic theories), which has the potential to transform the world's approach to economics and organizations of all sorts. As previously noted there is paradoxically always a scarcity of things, but at the same time an endless Abundance of possibilities. By tapping into everyone's inner source of vibrancy (i.e., the High Vibrational Energy sensibility of Abundance, Purpose and Possibility) in the context of a range of relationships (with self, other, group, Nature and Spirit) grounded in clarifying the agreements by which we can be, play and work together through processes and institutions, we can combine the simplicity of High Vibrancy relationships and clear agreements (strong "agreement fields") to create possibilities for ongoing transformation and regenerative flourishing individually and across our interconnected relationships and ecosystemic connections.

At a certain level of significant scale and complexity, which is for example (such as that inherent in the leadership and operation of global organizations, large cities, and states, and nation states), having at least Mature Integral capacities does matter. Ritchie-Dunham observes that in such complex settings while most of the engaged people need not be at the later stages of maturity such as Mature Integral, to optimize capacity and outcomes there needs to be something like a circle of active advisors who are.

The influence of the theory and initiatives of Wilber, Scharmer and Ritchie-Dunham have been spreading rapidly and transformatively across the globe. There are not many Kosmic Patterning Aware or later initiatives or leadership yet, because such people currently represent a miniscule percentage of humanity. Yet even though only a small number of such initiatives and leaders exist or are likely to be emerging soon, their influence for flourishing is already having a global impact.

The YOUnify Initiative[47], which I co-founded and chair is working with these sensibilities. YOUNify, is a societal transformation initiative co-founded and chaired by the author, which is grounded in IPP principles. It has the goal of creating interrelated individual, community and ecosystemic flourishing primarily by bridging divides of all sorts and making progress on the pressing issues of our time with multi-sectoral and multi-generational approaches. But we often say that are engaged more deeply in working with wounded and fractured people in wounded and fractured societies to heal together is a spirit of Sacred Wholeness as we experience the beauty of inspired solutions arising out of our shared Oneness.

YOUnify supports capacity building of organizations and coalitions with similar goals providing training, coaching and consulting at the intersection of stakeholder engagement, community organizing and behavioral science including applying all the insights and applications of IPP described in this book. YOUnify supports place-based grass roots and grass-tops community organizing as well as facilitates a leaders network. It co-hosts self-organizing learning laboratories on topics on specific thematic areas such as health, mental health, and flourishing; and climate change, sustainability, and regenerative systems. YOUnify plays a leading role in various national initiatives in the United States, such as co-chairing the "America Talks" initiative in collaboration with USA Today, Google News and others. It is currently engaging in 40 states in the United States and six other countries. It is organized as a global action network and connects and synergizes with other action networks to encourage local-global communities of practice around learning, public policy, and action. YOUnify is particularly involved in helping to lead the global conversation regarding global flourishing goals taking the place of United Nations global sustainability goals.

Although they work with people at all stages of development an outstanding example of one of the few organizations which guide and support individuals explicitly in growing into and experiencing in a healthy and productive way the full spectrum of human development including inhabiting the Causal Tier with an emphasis on leadership is Pacific Integral led by Geoff Fitch and Abigail Lynam[48]. They provide programs, coaching, and training informed by the latest research on human development. Particularly impressive is their group cohort program called Generating Transformative Change (GTC). For more than 15 years through over twenty-nine programs delivered on three continents, GTC has developed into a profoundly powerful, awakening, and mature learning journey. In a group cohort setting GTC promotes a shared desire for individuals to transform themselves, their organizations, communities, and our human consciousness, motivated by a vision of a more beautiful, equitable and sustainable future for all. Participants are supported in awakening to new versions of self, relationship, systems, conception, innovation, and the spirit of love for the Whole. People complete GTC with more awareness, aliveness, and vision for their own roles as leaders for flourishing in bringing about positive evolution for planetary life and leave with the practical knowledge, skills, and a community of support, to help make their vision a reality[49].

The Still Point Virtue of Being of each subtle polarity and the Character Virtues that flow from it, occur naturally only in the Causal Tier of development. In this and other ways IPP practice over time is an attractor into this tier of development and is preparation for leading from the Causal Tier. There are IPP polarities aligned with each of the four stages of the Causal Tier but specifically addressing them is beyond the scope of this book. They are summarized in Schedule 2, the Polarity Overview of the Human World.

Through the IPP Institute, courses are offered on the IPP Causal Tier polarities, and I assess and mentor individuals who are living from somewhere within the Causal Tier on flourishing and leadership for flourishing. Brief descriptions of characteristics of people with developmental centers of gravity at each of the four stages in the Causal Tier are set forth in Schedule 5.

Just as practicing IPP Subtle Tier polarities is an attractor to the Causal Tier of development, practicing Causal Tier Polarities is an attractor to a projected Non-Dual Tier of four further post-polar stages of development. IPP includes practices which support growing into perhaps that last major tier of human evolution.

Schedules

Polarity Overview – Primal Polarities

	POLAR NAME	PRIMARY POLARITY
LIFE WORLD	**INTENTION**	Desire (Seeking) Aversion
	AWARENESS	focus open
	PERCEPTION	Out In
MATERIAL WORLD	**LIFE**	Contraction Expansion
	MANIFESTATION	Energy (Wave) Mass (Particle)
	REALITY	Consciousness Spirit
FOUNDATIONAL POLARITIES	**DIVINITY**	Divine Masculine Divine Feminine
	CREATION	Ascending Descending
	IDENTITY	Uniquely Personal Universally Divine

BEING VIRTUE POLAR GIFT	VIRTUES OF BECOMING / DOING / POLAR VIRTUE		
Full Sacred Intent	**B** **D** **V**	Gratitude Generosity Giving-Receiving	
Awake Sacred Light	**B** **D** **V**	Present Witnessing (Latest Perspective) Clarity-Confusion	
Open Sacred Love	**B** **D** **V**	Wonder (Humility) Beautiful Loving Creativity Creation - Destruction	
Serene Sacred Life	**B** **D** **V**	Acceptance (Savor) Connection with Life Force/Flow/ Vibrancy Life-Death	
Endless Manifestation Sacred Manifestation	**B** **D** **V**	Awe Connection/Kosmic Emergence Vibration-Primal Consciousness (Prehension)	
Wholeness of Reality Sacred Reality	**B** **D** **V**	Enlightened Light Clarity-Confusion	
Wholeness of Divinity Sacred Divinity	**B** **D** **V**	Loving Love Joy-Sorrow	
Wholeness of Creation Sacred Creation	**B** **D** **V**	Vibrancy Life Permanence-Impermanence	
Wholeness of Identity Sacred Unique Expression	**B** **D** **V**	Reverence Unique Compassionate Embrace Love-Freedom	

Polarity Overview – Human World

		POLAR NAME	PRIMARY POLARITY
CAUSAL TIER	6.5	**KOSMIC INTEGRATIVE PURPOSE**	locus/ worlds
	6.0	**KOSMOS AWARE**	endless space-time/ spaceless-timeless
	5.5	**KOSMIC PATTERNING**	witnessing / kosmic patterns
	5.0	**CONSTRUCT AWARE**	language meaning/ empty language
SUBTLE TIER	4.5	INTEGRATIVE PURPOSE	integration/ reintegration
	4.0	CONTEXT AWARE	contextualization / deconstruction
	3.5	ACHIEVEMENT	subjectification/ objectification
	3.0	EXPERTISE	assert knowledge/ yield to knowledge
CONCRETE TIER	2.5	**PURPOSE**	facilitate (lead)/ inquire (follow)
	2.0	**MEANING**	alignment/ deviation
	1.5	**POWER**	control/ submission
	1.0	**RELATIONS**	agency/ communion

BEING VIRTUE POLAR GIFT	VIRTUES OF BECOMING / DOING / POLAR VIRTUE		
Kosmic Luminous Mind Sacred Kosmic Mind	**B** **D** **V**	Kosmic Presence Kosmic Light Kosmic Clarity/Confusion	
Kosmic Not-Twoness Sacred Kosmic Heart	**B** **D** **V**	Kosmic Hope Kosmic Love Kosmic Joy/Sorrow	
Kosmic Equanimity Sacred Kosmic Creation	**B** **D** **V**	Kosmic Accpetance Kosmic Life Kosmic Birth/Death	
Kosmic Silence Sacred Kosmic Engagement	**B** **D** **V**	Kosmic Reverence Kosmic Unique Embrace Kosmic Freedom/Love	
One Sacred Integration	**B** **D** **V**	Authenticity Harmony Spontaneous/Composed	
Whole Sacred Ecology	**B** **D** **V**	Sensitive Inclusive Same/Different	
Completion Sacred Accomplishment	**B** **D** **V**	Patient Effortless Accomplishment Beginning/Ending	
Quiet Mind Sacred Knowledge	**B** **D** **V**	Open Minded Light Realization/Illusion	
Fulfilled Sacred Flourishing	**B** **D** **V**	Inspired Non Judgmental Judgment/No Judgment	
Perfect Sacred Perfection	**B** **D** **V**	Integrity Forgiveness Remember/Forget	
Peace Sacred Empowerment	**B** **D** **V**	Humility Inspired Influence Gentleness/Firmness	
Trust Sacred Joy	**B** **D** **V**	Hope Love Joy/Sorrow	

Non-Dual – Foundational Polarity Overview

NON-DUAL
TIER
INFERRED
PRIOR
POLARITIES

Yang/Yin

Evolution/Involution

Absolute/Relative

CAUSAL HUMAN WORLD

SUBTLE LIFE WORLD

CONCRETE MATERIAL WORLD

Consciousness/Spirit

Divine Masculine/Divine Feminine

Ascending/Descending

Universally Divine/Uniquely Personal

FOUNDA-
TIONAL
META
POLARITIES

Non-Dual Involutionary Practice

PERSPECTIVE	CAUSAL
FIRST PERSPECTIVE (AWARE / CAUSAL)	Awareness of Awareness
	Fullness / Emptiness
SECOND PERSPECTIVE (RELATIONAL / SUBTLE)	Awareness of We
	Witness / No Other
THIRD PERSPECTIVE (PHYSICAL / GROSS)	Awareness of It
	Ifinite SpaceTime / No SpaceTime
INTEGRATION (INTEGRATION)	Awareness of Integration
	Fully Integrated / No Integration

SUBTLE	GROSS
Beauty	Wisdom (Light)
Inspiration / Creation	Clarity / Confusion
Goodness	Compassion (Love)
Mercy / Justice	Joy / Sorrow
Truth	Energy (Life)
Objectivity / Subjectivity	Permanence / Impermanence
Unique Engagement	Passionate Embrace
Liberty / Responsibility	Love / Freedom

Brief Descriptions of the Four Stages of the Causal Tier of Development*

CONSTRUCT AWARE

People with a developmental center of gravity at Construct Aware experience a dramatically new sense of identity due to stepping into a whole new tier of development. This new identity is grounded in causal awareness, which is deeper than the processing of the subtle thinking mind. Experiencing the emergence of this new sense of self can be profoundly disorienting. One can see more clearly from this altitude of development that words and language are constructed, that the narratives of our lives are constructs, as are the boundaries and guidelines in our cultural and societal environments. It is helpful for people at this stage of development to find qualified mentors, guides, and therapists who understand that this is merely the beginning of another tier of development rather than some kind of breakdown, since there is little understanding of this stage or of the Causal Tier in society at large even in the therapeutic community.

KOSMIC PATTERNING AWARE

A person at Kosmic Patterning Aware can recognize patterns that enable them to discern how philosophies, sciences, arts, and perspectives of all sorts can be interconnected and integrated in ways that are beyond the capacities of the subtle thinking mind. One tends to orient towards global and multi-generational concerns even as a sense of the preciousness of each moment is deepened. People at this stage tend to be active and engaged in making a difference due to their enhanced ability to manage complexity and to create, plan, and accomplish so much.

KOSMOS AWARE

The profoundly deep patterning that so engrosses those at Kosmic Patterning Aware is seen to be empty in a way to those at Kosmic Aware, as one opens to the vastness of a more Kosmic experience, of being in reciprocity with all of manifestation. Even space and time can be seen to be constructs, as they are experienced without any limits and are themselves empty. One often experiences the whole Kosmos flowing through oneself, particularly the quality of unlimited Love and Compassion for self, others, and all life and Being. The high energy assertiveness of Kosmic Patterning Aware tends to be subsumed in an overwhelming experience of the vastness of all manifestation, the emptiness of awareness, and intimations of Non-Duality.

KOSMIC INTEGRATIVE PURPOSE

As one moves into the Kosmic Integrative Purpose Stage there is a deep and active quality of developmental integration as well as passive Acceptance of all that arises. This developmental integration tends to take into account the full developmental range of manifestation: the concrete World of Matter, the subtle Life World, and the causal Human World, through the billions of years of emergence of the Kosmos. The emptiness of awareness and the fullness of all manifestation begin to interpenetrate, as do the poles of any locus of personal identity and of all manifestation.

As with the rest of the Human World stages and related IPP polarities, for the Causal Tier I have aligned stages of development and related IPP polarities with the Stages model of human development, but I use my own terminology for those stages to align with other IPP terminology more fully. There is no universal agreement among ego development theorists on the number and nature of stages of development beyond Mature Integral. However, I was one of four people involved in the original scoring research for the Causal Tier in the Stages model, and over the years have observed that even as characterizations of these stages continue to evolve based on ongoing practice and scoring research, the stages themselves have had enduring integrity—always keeping in mind that every model is a map and not the territory.

Notes

1.   For additional information about and resources for learning and practicing integral polarity practice, see the website of the Integral Polarity Practice Institute, www.theippinstitute.com.

2.   Ken Wilber, a leading philosopher of human development and the founder of the integral school of philosophy, with a deep grasp of the traditions of both East and West, has noted: "There is nobody doing more leading-edge work on the integration of Eastern and Western approaches to consciousness and growth than John Kesler. His fully integral approach includes conventional and contemplative dimensions of psychology and spirituality, spanning body, mind, spirit, and shadow, a truly remarkable and effective approach." IPP Institute, accessed February 24, 2024, https://theippinstitute.com/.

3.   Much research supports the idea that Love is the most important principle of flourishing. See for instance the chapter by Matthew T. Lee, PhD, then director of Empirical Research at the Institute for Quantitative Research for the Harvard Human Flourishing Program, "Love as the Essence of Flourishing: Educational Experiments with the Subjunctive Mood," in *The Future of Education: Reimagining Its Aims and Responsibilities*, ed. Jonathan Beale and Christina Easton (New York: Oxford University Press, 2024), chap. 3.

4.   Words that represent transcendent qualities are capitalized throughout.

5.   Transcendent and Divine are used interchangeably in this book.

6.   Mamie Payne, LCSW, therapist, certified IPP facilitator, and IPP teacher candidate notes: "Engaging the whole person from a systems approach and following a developmentally-informed perspective along the continuum of the human lifespan, the IPP framework offers unique precision in both the identification and pointed repair of early core attachment wounds and other maladaptive internal holdings that inhibit trusting connections and diminish optimal biopsychosocial spiritual functioning. IPP as a practice framework and diagnostic tool enables a process that I have begun to refer to as *meta-attachment*, in that it reliably fosters experiential reconnection and somatic co-regulation with a boundless source of connective and healing energy that transcends normal aspects of personality and the ego, and in process offers individualized insights into how to quiet the conflict of the mind, and repair attachment wounds that have been incurred along a lifetime of human development." Email dated August 29, 2022.

7.   Terri O. Fallon, PhD, a leading researcher and theorist in the school of ego development in developmental psychology and leader of Stages International and Developmental Research Institute, has noted: "There are many approaches and practices to awareness and how one manifests in the world that can serve humanity's trek along the journey of waking up and growing up, but I am not aware of any applied practice which covers the entire developmental continuum in this regard other than John Kesler's IPP practice. It is unique; no matter where you are along the continuum of growing up, he has corresponding practices to support both your 'waking up' and your 'growing up.'" "Who We Are," IPP Institute, accessed February 24, 2024, https://theippinstitute.com/about.

8.   Identifying the Still Points of key universal, archetypal polarities related to stages of human development is a unique contribution of IPP. Susanne Cook-Greuter, PhD, one of the most prominent researchers and theorists of human development in this generation, has observed: "John Kesler has created the richest matrix that covers development through the whole spectrum of consciousness from birth through personal individuation into the heart of Big Mind. Kesler provides exquisite detail within an elegant and comprehensive structure. His polarity map illuminates the still points between polar opposites at multiple developmental junctures along the way. By clarifying just what the fundamental tensions are, he has deepened our understanding of

human development and experience in a profound way." "Who We Are," IPP Institute.

9.   In this stage of polar maturity, both poles are being held and then one swings back and forth in a double looping pattern to alternate which pole is optimally emphasized in the moment. It is reflected in the theory and work of Barry Johnson and his concept of polarity management. A developmental approach to this same polarity dynamic has been developed by Beena Sharma with Dr. Cook-Greuter through the Vertical Development Academy. See Polarity Partnerships, https://www.polaritypartnerships.com, and Vertical Development Academy, https://verticaldevelopment.com.

10.   Voice dialogue is a Jungian therapeutic technique, whereby you speak to and from aspects of the self. The author was originally trained in using voice dialogue as a teaching modality to support others in accessing transcendent qualities when he was one of the first people to become approved to facilitate large groups in the Zen Big Mind Process developed by Genpo Roshi.

11.   The terms "concrete," "subtle," and "causal" are derived from the Vedantic tradition and are used regularly in many commentaries on meditation with reference to primary qualities of awareness. These terms are used more generally here as referring to any spectrum that designates three degrees of refinement that can be referred to in multiple ways—i.e., extremely concrete, to concrete, to less concrete; or not very refined, to refined, to very refined. One way or another the reference relates to dividing a spectrum of granularity into three categories. The "causal" category traditionally refers to peak refinement and Stillness. In IPP we use the "concrete," "subtle," "causal" terminology in multiple dimensions and applications to identify a common harmonic among multiple aspects. When doing this you discover that there are resonating relationships among aspects that may not otherwise seem to share commonalities, such as "states of awareness" and "stages of development." In the context of IPP practice we hold states and stages as harmonic expressions of the same underlying qualities. You must stabilize in a "state" before a "stage" with those same qualities can emerge. That is necessary but not sufficient for a stage to emerge. For instance, one can stabilize in causal meditative capacities in the Subtle Tier of development but still not have emerged into the Causal Tier of development. Clearly there is much more to say about this topic than is possible here.

12.   For our purposes here, there is just one polarity for the Concrete World. In many ways the IPP framework and patterns are adjusted to accommodate an emphasis on meaningful practice rather than trying to create full consistency, for instance in terms of numbers of stages in a "tier" or a "world."

13.   The question might be asked how there can be stages of Non-Duality, when Non-Duality is a quality beyond any expression, description, or hierarchy. The answer is that these are four stages of human development that are projected to emerge once one has developmentally and structurally grown into a stabilized Non-Dual realization developmentally beyond the Causal Tier. Many meditative traditions stabilize practitioners in Non-Duality, but in the context of developmental psychology, that has essentially amounted in most cases to a stabilized "state" rather than a fully realized structural "stage." It appears that historically very few people have grown into the Non-Dual structural stages of Development, although due to recently developed practices that take into consideration human stage development, such as IPP, increasing numbers of people may begin growing into that developmental Tier. The Stages model of human development projects four developmental stages in what it calls the Unified Tier of human development, based on its projections of iterating patterns of human development. IPP aligns itself with the Stages model and its many iterating patterns, including this projected tier of development referred to here as the Non-Dual Tier, but the themes expressed on the IPP chart for this tier, and which are echoed in the four Foundational Polarities, are sourced solely from the author's

intuition.

14.   The IPP Harmonic is merely a construct, as is the entire IPP practice ecosystem. On the other hand, IPP touches into many patterns that seem to resonate well with life and reality and is specifically designed to provide a user-friendly harmonic and practice framework in service of flourishing.

15.   IPP master teacher Thomas McConkie, who has significant training in multiple meditative traditions, has led many weeklong IPP meditation retreats introducing IPP through focusing significantly on the Life Tier Polarities. To date Thomas is the sole full successor to the author as an IPP master teacher. He is currently attending Harvard Divinity School, writing a thesis on integral polarity practice as a new model for human development and transformation.

16.   See the Presencing Institute website, u-school for Transformation, https://www.u-school.org.

17.   Keith J. Karren, N. Lee Smith, and Kathryn J. Gordon, *Mind Body Health: The Effects of Attitudes, Emotions, and Relationships*, 5th ed. (San Francisco: Pearson Education, 2014), chaps. 2, 4–6, 11–14, 15–17, and summary, pp. 447–49. One of the coauthors of the book, N. Lee Smith, MD, a certified IPP facilitator, has stated, "IPP practice enhances the primary principles of human flourishing in the very foundational polarities it considers. One *experiences* these principles with IPP. I know of no other meditative practice that addresses all these as directly." Email dated February 26, 2024

NOTES PART II

18.   See, for example, John McKnight and Peter Block, *Abundant Community: Awakening the Power of Families and Neighborhoods* (San Francisco: Berrett-Koehler, 2010).

19.   Daniel P. Brown and David S. Elliott, *Attachment Disturbances in Adults: Treatment for Comprehensive Repair* (New York: W.W. Norton, 2016). Professor Brown was also a leading scholar, translator, and teacher relating to Tibetan Buddhist and related Indigenous Bon meditative traditions. He noticed that meditators would have significant difficulties on the meditative path if they suffered from attachment disorders relating to the absence of any of these positive principles of healthy attachment in their childhood. Accordingly, he developed corrective therapeutic approaches aligned with findings of the above publication.

20.   See, for example, consistent references herein to the work of James Ritchie-Dunham, Matthew Lee, and particularly Katy Granville-Chapman and Emmie Bidston.

21.   This is a brief description of the well-known "four quadrants of knowledge" model framed by integral philosopher Ken Wilber, and it is also reflected in the work of James Ritchie-Dunham. For various reasons these Four Primary Dimensions are often included in training related to the Relations Polarity. They are embedded in the IPP framework. There is also some ambiguity here as to whether a group with a defined purpose is serving a broader ecosystem all the way from supply lines to customers, for instance, or whether the group itself is defined as the ecosystem. Rather than being precise here it is important to appreciate that every group and organization is an ecosystem in the context of other ecosystems, but may or may not be defined as such for purposes being addressed.

22.   When the poles, systemization/re-systemization (also integration/reintegration), fully flow into one another, one begins to emerge into not only the next stage of development but the next "tier" of development. From this new perspective one begins to see how the subtle thinking mind's capacity to systematize is limited in what it can meaningfully embrace—i.e., endless complex adaptive systems within systems, systemically connected to other systems within

system, etc.— and is transcended (albeit included in) by the patterning capacities of the "causal" awareness in that next Causal Tier of development.

23.   IPP emphasizes the importance of the pervasive presence of Love in one's relationships with the Transcendent (God, Divine, Spirit, Source, Ultimate, Absolute, Higher Self—however one defines that), self, others, groups, etc., and our life world as the essence of flourishing. Note that Love is frequently clustered with the transcendent qualities of Light and Life, usually in the progression of Light, Love, and Life. The author assumes that these three qualities are different resonances of the same Essence or Spirit, but this framing and its implications for a richer framing of the essence of flourishing are not developed in this book.

24.   The broader vision here is an appreciation of the ecosystemic reality of all manifestation, from the sub-atomic level through the cosmic scale, with humanity being one interconnected ecosystemic dimension of this. From this perspective, it helps us develop the sense of our stewardship for the integrity and flourishing of the ecosystems, of which we are composed and of which we are a part.

25.   Matthew T. Lee and Isha Mayor, "Health and Flourishing: An Interdisciplinary Synthesis," in *Human Flourishing: A Multidisciplinary Perspective on Neuroscience, Health, Organizations and Arts*, ed. Mireia Las Heras, Marc Grau-Grau, and Yasin Rofcanin (Cham, Switzerland: Springer, 2023), 49–68.

26.   James Ritchie-Dunham with Bettye Pruitt, *Ecosynomics: The Science of Abundance* (Belchertown, MA: Vibrancy Publishing, 2014), 38–41.

27.   Based on considerable research, the Stages model describes how when one grows into a new sense of subtle individuality in Early and then Mature Modern stages of development, the collective that you identify with (particularly at Early Modern), or are at least fully familiar with, is still the traditional collective. See Stages descriptions in this regard at Stages International, www.stagesinternational.com.

28.   Tyler J. VanderWeele, "On the Promotion of Human Flourishing," PNAS 114, no. 31 (2017): 8148–56.

29.   Matthew T. Lee, Molly Hartsough, Sam Borick, and Brooks Gathagan, "Open Space, Transformative Education, and the Pursuit of Flourishing," *Journal of Transformative Education* 19, no. 3 (2021): 198–217.

30.   The transcendent poles that flow out of Unique Compassionate Embrace are Love and Freedom—the ultimate high value outputs of the IPP involutionary trajectory.

31.   A framing developed by Thich Nhat Hanh. See his book *Interbeing: Fourteen Guidelines for Engaged Buddhism*, rev. ed. (Berkeley, CA: Parallax Press 1998). Another framing, "intra-being," has appeared more recently in various settings inferring an underlying quality of Oneness.

32.   The other most prominent triumvirate of Virtues of Becoming, Doing and Being are Gratitude and Generosity arising out of Abundance.

33.   Ed Brooks, "Practicing the Art of Good Hope," Oxford Pastorate, June 26, 2018, https://oxfordpastorate.org/news/practising-the-art-of-good-hope.

34.   The Oxford Character Project, https://oxfordcharacter.org.

35.   Tyler J. VanderWeele, "Why Caring and Character Matter," Psychology Today, December 21, 2022, https://www.psychologytoday.com/us/blog/human-flourishing/202212/why-caring-and-character-matter.

36.   Katy Granville-Chapman and Emmie Bidston, *Leader: Know, Love and Inspire Your People* (Carmarthen, Wales: Crown House Publishing, 2020).

37.   Supported by the author's observations of these two women in action.

38.   Verónica Fernández Espinosa, "The Effect of Teacher Leadership on Students'

Purposeful Learning," *Cogent Social Sciences* 9, no. 1 (2023), available online at https://www.tandfonline.com/doi/full/10.1080/23311886.2023.2197282.

39. An implication of the high impact of voice dialogue with those at Early Integral and later is that sharing IPP through voice dialogue tends to be less impactful for those at stages of development earlier than Early Integral.

40. Note the important work being done by Professor Amos Guiora to criminalize enabling of serious abuse and bystanders failing to report serious abuse: Amos N. Guiora, *Armies of Enablers: Survivor Stories of Complicity and Betrayal in Sexual Assaults* (Chicago: American Bar Association, 2020). Note also a description of the Bystanders Initiative led by Professor Guiora: Suzi Morales, "New Initiative Studies 'Ecosystem' of Abuse," S.J. Quinney College of Law, University of Utah, January 4, 2023, https://sjquinney.utah.edu/news-articles/new-initiative-studies-ecosystem-of-abuse/. The author is personally engaged in promoting this work.

41. As another summary of the IPP Harmonic discussed in the "Deeper IPP Patterns, Structures, and Practices" section of Part I, the base IPP harmonic is composed of the following themes or "notes": "ground, concrete, subtle, causal, and integration," which are pervasive in IPP. For instance, there are the thematic tiers of development in the IPP ecosystem: The Life Tier is the Ground Tier of the Human World. The Human World comprises the Concrete Tier, the Subtle Tier, and Causal Tier. There is a projected fully integrated Non-Dual Tier of the Human World. The top or integrative stages of each tier is the ground stage that gives birth to the stages of the next tier. For instance, the Intent Polarity, which is the integrative stage of the Concrete Tier, is also the ground polarity of the first Concrete Tier of the Human World, which is composed of concrete, subtle, causal, and integrative polar stages, etc.

42. Quote drawn from an unpublished paper by Mami Ishii, ND, entitled "Japanese Delicious Moment Therapy; An Integration of Traditional Japanese Aesthetic Healing into Psychotherapy." See also Mami Ishii and Ted Lo, "Oishii: Delicious Moment Therapy," in *Asian Healing Traditions in Counseling and Psychotherapy*, ed. Roy Moodley, Ted Lo, and Na Zhu (Los Angeles: Sage Publications, 2018), chap. 17.

43. The author has had the privilege of being acquainted with Ramona Sierra and her work for many years.

44. Healing Conversations Conference: Toward Bridging Social and Political Divisions, Utah Valley University, March 30, 2023.

45. C. Otto Scharmer, *Theory U: Leading from the Future as It Emerges* (San Francisco: Berrett-Koehler Publishers, 2009).

46. Ritchie-Dunham, *Ecosynomics*.

47. See the YOUnify website, www.younify.org.

48. Pacific Integral, www.pacificintegral.com.

49. Following are some groups that provide training for personal and leadership development that explicitly supports people in moving beyond Mature Integral: Integral Life which explicitly supports Ken Wilber's theory and vision; Center for Leadership Maturity and Vertical Development Academy led by Suzanne Cook-Greuter and Beena Sharma; and Stages International led by Terri O'Fallon. Lower Lights School of Wisdom (www.lowerlightswisdom.org), led by Thomas McConkie and Gloria Pak, provides a unique, millennial approach to participating in spiritual community in the context of spiritual deepening and human development.

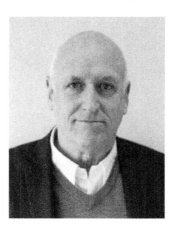

JOHN KESLER formulated a spiritual, life and societal transformation practice framework known as integral polarity practice ("IPP") and has shared IPP for over twenty years through the IPP Institute (www.theippinstitute.com). John speaks, teaches, and consults through the lens of IPP in service of greater interrelated individual, collective, and ecosystemic flourishing and leadership for flourishing. He may be contacted at john@theippinstitute.com.

John graduated from Columbia University Law School in 1973 and continues to practice law. He was a founding member of the politics section of the Integral Institute founded by Ken Wilber. John served as executive director of the United States Coalition of Healthy Cities and Communities, and as co-chair of the Healthy Communities Global Action Network. He was communities editor of the National Civic Review.

John is co-founder and chair of YOUnify, a non-profit initiative grounded in IPP principles and dedicated to bridging differences of all sorts in service of interrelated individual, collective, and ecosystemic flourishing (www.younify.org). He is a member of the Harvard/Oxford interest group on Leadership for Flourishing and chair of the civic and government committee of the Spirituality and Flourishing interest group, both part of the Harvard University Flourishing Network ("HFN"). He leads an HFN Community of Practice dedicated to promoting flourishing and transformation primarily through applications of IPP. John is a fellow of the Institute for Strategic Clarity.

Printed in Great Britain
by Amazon

42176312R00076